Atkins Diet For Beginners

A Simple Way of Eating That Automatically Allows You to Lose Weight and Feel Great.

Modern Meals Plans Included

Michael D. Kaiser

Published by:

Dana Publishing
P.O. Box 1801
Mentor, OH 44060

Legal & Disclaimer

Upon using the contents and information contained in this book, you agree to hold harmless the Author from and against any damages, costs, and expenses, including any legal fees potentially resulting from the application of any of the information provided by this book. This disclaimer applies to any loss, damages or injury caused by the use and application, whether directly or indirectly, of any advice or information presented, whether for breach of contract, tort, negligence, personal injury, criminal intent, or under any other cause of action.

You agree to accept all risks of using the information presented inside this book.

You agree that by continuing to read this book, where appropriate and/or necessary, you shall consult a professional (including but not limited to your doctor, attorney, or financial advisor or such other advisor as needed) before using any of the suggested remedies, techniques, or information in this book.

Table of Contents

Introduction

The Atkins Diet is one of the most popular diets of all time with millions of people around the world claiming that it has made a difference in their life. It focuses on increasing the amount of protein that you consume, along with reducing your carb intake. The primary focus of the diet has to do with being hypersensitive to carbohydrates that are problematic. By reducing carbohydrates, our weight should also reduce, or, at least, that is the theory.

The Atkins Diet is now seeing resurgence as many experts are looking at this diet in a new way. If done correctly, this diet plan can be a healthy life style change. Yes, a healthy life, plus a new way to look at food. You can view the Atkins Diet as your way to shed those extra pounds you cannot seem to shake off no matter what exercise or diet you have tried. Sometimes, it seems like no matter what you do, you just cannot achieve the ideal body that you want. The Atkins Diet is your solution.

For those of you that are looking to lose more than just five or ten pounds, the Atkins Diet will allow you to lose a large amount of weight in just the first two to three weeks, with no strenuous exercise necessary. Your body itself will be doing all the work for you. The rest is learning how to keep the weight off and continue to eat healthy. This, in turn, will help you keep those extra pounds off for life.

We can look at the Atkins Diet as a new beginning in properly eating to become more healthy. When you research and learn more about the Atkins Diet, it is safe and actually gives you the results you want. We first need to come to the conclusion that our enemy is the carbohydrates and not the fats. If we eat the right carbs in the right amounts, we can lose weight and keep it off for good.

Why Carbs Are Bad for You

Carbohydrates are the main source of energy for our bodies. Athletes need carbs to perform well and keep their energy up, meaning that the Atkins diet is seemingly impossible for those types of people. For the average person, the problem occurs when the carbs you are in taking come from a sugary, fatty coffee early in the morning. A small amount of the carbohydrates are used for energy, while the remainder is stored as fat deposits for later use.

Our bodies have this primeval programming that someday, we might be left in a desert and will need to store energy in the form of fat for future use. Sadly, the body over compensates and stores more fat than we need. We are consuming far more sugar than our body is able to process and that is the main problem. When the body is presented with fats and sugars, it takes the body more energy to burn fats we consume than to use the available sugars that we have consumed prior.

Chapter 1: About the Atkins Diet

If truth be told right now, you've probably tried diet after diet with little to no success. If you haven't actually been on a diet before, then you must know someone that has. Most diets around require you to count calories and many will require that you avoid foods high in fat. However, there's one particular diet that is very popular and does not require you to do either of those things. In fact, you can eat as much as you'd like of eggs, red meat, bacon, cheese and butter!

As with any other popular diet, and especially with a diet that allows you to eat so many foods that are generally off limits with diets, the Atkins Diet has received much controversy. However, various studies show that the Atkins Diet can help result in weight loss and is actually better than a number of other diets. Not to mention the fact that dieters all over the world are satisfied with the weight loss results that they've achieved with Atkins.

The Atkins Diet is one of the most popular diets out there. It focuses on reducing the intake of carbohydrates while incorporating protein-rich foods. Most of us eat more carbohydrates than anything else in a day, which consists of refined sugar and white flour. In other words, your favorite foods, such as cereal, bread and pasta, contain a large amount of carbohydrates. By limiting your carb intake, you are forcing your body into a state in which it must burn stored fat rather than carbs for fuel.

As already explained, you do need to watch how many carbs are consumed each day; however, there's no need to count calories – which can get a bit mind-numbing when dieting.

So, why do you have to count carbs but not calories? Well, Dr. Atkins, the creator of the Atkins Diet, has performed vigorous research and countless experimentations to come to the conclusion that too many carbohydrates – not too much fat – is actually the main cause of weight gain in individuals. Primarily, this is because when too many carbs enter the body, insulin levels soar triggering fat storage.

How You Lose Weight on the Atkins Diet

At the Atkins Diet focuses on the restriction of carbohydrates. When the body is unable to convert carbs into fuel, it will turn to other methods of creating fuels. With the Atkins Diet, your body will use fat for fuel rather than carbohydrates. Therefore, when consuming little to no carbohydrates, the body's fat storage will thus became its primary source of energy.

In order to really understand how the Atkins Diet helps you lose weight, let's look at how the body creates fuel from sugar. For sugar to be converted into fuel, insulin must be used. Controlling how much sugar is in our blood, insulin makes it possible for the cells in our bodies to turn carbs into glucose. Insulin is secreted to avoid soaring, out of control blood sugar levels. Because insulin is a hormone of storage, sugar that is not converted to fuel will be stored as fat. At the same time, insulin is what keeps the body from efficiently burning stored fat.

According to the Atkins Diet, it is that insulin response that keeps us from losing weight and continuing to add more and more fat to the body. When we have little food, this can be a good thing; however, high-carb and sugar-filled foods will only cause us to accumulate more body fat.

In contract, a low-carb diet will encourage less insulin production. According to the Atkins Diet and various resources online, when your body can maintain a normal insulin level, the body turns to its own fat to convert into fuel. This process results in weight loss. If insulin levels can be kept stable, the body will burn fat and will likely lead to fewer cravings and a suppressed appetite.

So, in a nutshell, the Atkins Diet helps you lose weight by putting you on a very low-carb diet that will help control insulin levels.

The Four Phases of the Atkins Diet

There are four phases in the Atkins Diet: induction, ongoing weight loss, pre-maintenance and maintenance. The duration of each of these phases varies per individual. Atkins now says that you do not have to start with the first phase, but it is recommended since it will give your weight loss efforts a huge boost – even if you can't handle the first phase for the full two weeks that is advised. As you move forward with each phase, you will begin to slowly increase your carb intake while avoiding refined sugars and grains. Here's a more in-depth look at each phase, including information on the recommended length of the phase, what you can eat, and the primary goals of that particular phase in your weight loss efforts.

<u>Phase #1 – Induction</u>

This is the most restrictive phase of the diet and it is crucial that you follow this phase to the t. During this phase, which lasts for 14 days, you are allowed to eat very little, if any, carbohydrates. Essentially, you cannot consume more than 20 grams of carbs per day while in the induction phase. The carbs that can be consumed include low-carb, non-starchy vegetables. You can't eat fruits, grains, bread or certain dairy products during the first two weeks of the Atkins Diet.

Ultimately, this first phase is a way to jump-start your weight loss. Although the typical duration is two weeks, you may stay in the first phase for an extra week or so, if you choose, depending on the amount of weight loss you have had towards the end of this phase and your goal weight.

This phase's primary goal is to really get your weight loss journey started with rapid weight loss. When this happens, dieters often feel they are finally doing something right and have a little extra confidence that dieting really can help them lose weight. The induction phase also stabilizes your blood sugar levels, which will minimize, and possibly eliminate, your food cravings. However, keep in mind that you could also experience some mood swings and fatigue from the reduction in carbs and change in your body.

<u>Phase #2 – Ongoing Weight Loss</u>

The second phase gives you the chance to increase the amount of carbs you consume on a daily basis by five grams. You will take this phase week by week, increasing your carb intake by five grains each week. So, it will look like this:

☐   Week 1: 25 grams of carbs

☐   Week 2: 30 grams of carbs

☐   Week 3: 35 grams of carbs

☐   And so on.

You will continue to slowly increase your intake of carbohydrates until the time when your body hits a plateau and stops losing weight. At this point, you will want to subtract five grams of carbs from your diet each day. This will allow you to maintain your weight. This phase should carry on as long as needed to reach your weight loss goals. Depending on your individual metabolism, you'll consume anywhere from 25 to about 50 carbs per day.

The number of carbohydrates that you can eat while still losing weight is called your Critical Carbohydrate Level for Losing (CCLL) and is one of the primary goals of the Ongoing Weight Loss phase. It has also been developed to help you continue losing weight safely while also learning to consume new foods and limiting your carb intake so that you can still reduce your appetite and cravings.

Phase #3 – Pre-Maintenance

When you hit phase three, your main goal won't be to lose weight, but to maintain it instead. You won't enter this phase until you are within a few pounds of your goal weight – at least 10 pounds. You can increase your carb intake by 10 grams every week as long as you don't start gaining the weight back. Alternatively, you can yourself a nice treat every two or three days by consuming a 20-30 gram carbohydrate item. When you start gaining, you'll need to decrease your carb intake and remain at a lower daily amount.

At this point in the Atkins Diet, the primary goal is to determine how many carbs you can consume on a daily basis without gaining any weight. You will continue to lose weight, but at a much a slower pace, until you reach your final goal. This phase will also help you learn how you can maintain your weight moving forward.

Phase #4 – Lifetime Maintenance

The fourth and final phase of the Atkins Diet still limits your carbohydrate intake, but gives you a larger variety of foods to select from. This phase will help you ensure that the pounds you have lost do not come back while giving you more freedom when it comes to what you eat.

You will have to ensure you keep the bad, refined carbs out of your diet and only take in healthy carbs. As long as you pull together everything that you have learned thus far while on the Atkins Diet, you should have no problem successfully keeping your weight off since you know now your body's limit when it comes to carbohydrates. Most people will find that the right amount of carbs is between 75 and 100 grams of carbs per day.

Ultimately, at this point in time, you've reached your goal weight and are ready to move forward with your life in a new, improved and sexy body!

Chapter 2: Why the Big Deal About Carbohydrates

This will be a brief lesson on human metabolism for those people who are not medically inclined. I promise I will make this quick. Almost all foods can fall into three simple categories or a combination of them. There are the carbohydrates which can be found in grains, root type vegetables and fruits. Then there are the proteins which come mostly from meats such as beef, fish and chicken, as well as, some grains and vegetables, like certain seeds, nuts and beans. And finally, there are types of fats which can come from both plants and animals. For example, there is the animal fat in bacon that comes from pigs and coconut oil or olive oil which is both plant-derived. Now what is so important about this? By knowing this small bit of information, you can get an idea of where these sources come from and as we will discuss later, know the foods to consume and which to stay away from.

What are the carbohydrates for?

Carbohydrates are the main source of energy for our bodies to function. In order for a runner to complete a marathon, they had to consume some form of carbohydrate that the body converted to simple sugars which can be absorbed and converted into usable energy. The problem comes when that carbohydrate happens to be a sugary fatty rich coffee in the morning. A small amount of the carbohydrates are used for energy, the remainder is stored as fat deposits for future use.

Our bodies have this primeval programming that someday we will be left in some desert and will need to store energy in the form of fat for future use. Unfortunately, the body, as in many other processes in our body, over compensates and stores more than we would like. We are consuming far more sugar than our body is able to process and therefore has to store wherever it can. When the body is presented with the fats and sugar, it takes the body more energy to burn fats we consume than to use the readily available sugars that we consume. So as you can see, carbohydrates are not our friend after all.

Proteins:

Proteins are very extremely important as it is used for even the most basic functions in the human body. Proteins are what make up our very own strands of DNA, as well as our muscles and organs. A steady intake of lean protein is vital to weight loss, as the body will break down muscle first before breaking down your own stored fat for energy. Later, we will discuss that the eating of protein in our diet is very important so that the body will burn our fat and not breakdown muscle for energy.

Dr. Atkins' Diet Revolution:

When Doctor Atkins published his revolutionary diet ideas in his 1972 book title "Diet Revolution", it was received with plenty of skepticism and controversy. His idea did not align with those of the main stream medical community. As some years went by and people began to see success with his diet, the medical community then took notice and started conduct studies and documenting their own findings on this way of eating. As the message got out, Doctor Atkins' diet gained popularity in the early 2000s. One in eleven people in America were on the Atkins diet. But as the diet popularity grew, so did the negative propaganda. Some expert say it was started by the leaders of the carb industry who saw sales dropping at dramatic rates and people all over the western world were reminded about 'the dangers of fat'. Sadly after Dr Atkins passing from a head injury, the popularity of the diet began to see a declined.

The Atkins Diet Today:

But today, many health experts from around the world are calling to departments of health to quickly change their advice, amend the carbohydrate myth and tell people to eat a low-carb diet instead of a low fat one. Most diets tend to fail because you are constantly being told to curb your calories thus reducing the bulk of food you eat and thus feeling hungry all the time. With the Atkins diet, we are only reducing the carbohydrate intake. With the Atkins diet program, we are not counting calories; we are counting the amount or grams of carbohydrates you can eat. Thus, you can eat more and not feel constantly hungry.

Sugar not only causes weight gain but it is also highly addictive and causes a number of dangerous diseases that damage the body and affect how the brain functions like during a sugar rush. With our brain being made of 60% fat and the persistent trend towards cutting back on fats perhaps it is no surprise that the elderly seem to be suffering from more degenerative brain diseases than ever before. Later, we will discuss why this may be shown to be true in the future. It is also no wonder we are seeing more and more case of brain disorders in this country. The World Health Organization predicts that by 2040, as the populations get older, diseases such as Alzheimer's, dementia, Parkinson's disease, will overtake cancer to become the second leading cause of death after cardiovascular disease.

However, as Doctor Atkins said himself, 'this isn't a license to gorge'. There are still things to consider and steps to take to turn your body into a healthy fat-burning machine.

This introduction to the Atkins diet will guide you through each of the four phases to show you how to lose weight fast, keep it off and have a healthier body and mind all around. It will also tell you about some tasty low-carb recipes that will make your mouth absolutely water. In a nut shell, the Atkins diet is not just to lose weight, but a way of life.

Chapter 3: Why the Atkins Diet Will Work For You

It is a perfect diet for fast-paced and busy lifestyles. You will lose weight without any exercise. Your body will be doing all the work for you. If you do not follow the Atkins Diet strictly, you will not lose weight. There is no calorie counting, nor strict exercise regimens in the Atkins diet. Committing to the Atkins Diet does not take time out of your daily routine; rather, it is a change in your way of eating. All that is asked of you in this diet is to stick to the diet plan as strictly as possible. Eventually the types of foods that you can eat and in what quantities will become second nature and you will automatically know what to do.

But, imagine if we were to throw in a simple exercise plan that is not to elaborate but fits into your busy schedule. There are tons of options out there on the internet. Next time you are in front of the television, just take a second and look at all the different exercise options that are out there that you could consider for your fast-pace life. I happen to be a big Pinterest follower and I can tell you there is tons of information just on Pinterest. There are people just willing to provide us with their success stories on losing weight and how they did it and what exercise plan worked for them. But remember, with the Atkins diet, you will lose the weight without any exercise. But just imagine if you did add a small exercise plan to your daily routine. When you start to lose that weight fast and start to feel lighter and better all around, this is probably where you will consider exercising to intensify the weight loss.

Although I probably would not recommend exercising during the induction phase because the amount of carbohydrates that the body uses for energy is being restricted, I would on the other hand recommend waiting for one of the ladder phases since you will be more familiar with the diet plan and therefore, can focus on an exercise plan that will fit your schedule. The Atkins diet is basically knowing what you can and cannot eat and in what proportion of carbohydrates. You need to become a carb detective in everything you consume by reading every label.

The Benefits of The Atkins Diet:

<u>Increases Your Life Expectancy</u>

If you're having trouble committing to this healthy diet, pause for a moment and consider this. What would you give if someone offered to give you eight more years to your life? What would you be willing to pay? What would you do? Many studies have found a direct correlation between obesity and shorter life expectancy, by eight years. Shedding just 10 pounds can make your life longer, and better.

<u>Prevent A Heart Attack, Reduces Blood Pressure, And Prevents Diabetes:</u>

We are all probably tired of hearing and are very aware that obese individuals have a higher risk of heart disease, cancer, high blood pressure, breathing problems, Type II diabetes, and other conditions. For those with Type II diabetes, the Atkins Diet is one way to keep the diabetes under control. When you eat carbs, your body breaks them down into sugars. In Type II diabetes, there is too much sugar for the body's insulin to break down, which leads to some serious medical problems. If less carbs are consumed, there is less sugar in the blood, and the diabetes is under control. Imagine that; no more finger sticking to read blood sugar levels. No more having to inject yourself with insulin because your sugar levels will be low and the body will not require the insulin any more.

Even better, you will not have to deal with or at least prolong the long term effects of living with high levels of sugar in the blood. Some of these long term problems include loss of eye sight or an extremity in more extreme cases. Yes, losing a finger or two. The long term high sugar levels in the blood stream will cause the body to lose sensation to the hand, fingers and toes. If you were to hear yourself, you may not know it until it is too late. With the Atkins Diet, you will be eating a healthy diet and keeping the sugar levels down and hence reduces the possibility of having such complications.

The Atkins Diet also lowers the bad LDL cholesterol and raises the good HDL cholesterol. This diet has been studied extensively and there are studies now showing a lowering of bad cholesterol and an increase in the good cholesterol. Other studies related to the Atkins diet and even not related to the Atkins diet have shown a direct correlation between weight loss and a decrease in blood pressure for hypertensive patients. Yes, weight loss means lower blood pressure and a reduced risk of heart disease and atherosclerosis, and better heart health.

This healthy diet is not just about changing the way you look, but rather, a weight loss plan to help you live longer and healthier. That is why it is worth the commitment. We can go on with many more benefits of this diet on our health including mentioning of the effects of our current bad diet on the brain which is made up of about 60 percent fat. We should not be looking at just the immediate results of the diet but the long term effects on our health.

A Commitment to the Diet

Some popular diets say, "Hey, we know that our diet is so ridiculously difficult to follow, that we'll let you cheat (where you can break the diet and eat whatever you want) for one day/meal/whatever." But there are no cheat days in the Atkins Diet, because cheating doesn't work. If you break the diet and binge on carbs, you can add 1 to 5 pounds the next day. Although some of this is from retaining water (an effect of carb consumption), it may take up to a week to get back on track with your weight loss. Some people get nauseous and feel horrible when their carb levels spike. And sometimes, breaking the diet leads to super strong carb cravings, which make it even tougher to follow the diet. If you do mess up one day, do not give up. You can get right back on track. However, it is easier to just say "no" to those mashed potatoes at Thanksgiving dinner. Just be strong-willed. People will respect you more when they see the new and healthier you.

The Psychological Approach to Long-Term Weight Loss

Just because you're on a diet, doesn't mean you have to be miserable. You just need to make some adjustment to the way you approach your meals. If you're a pasta lover, find low-carb vegetable pastas. As mentioned earlier, I will provide you with some resources to low-carb recipes that you are accustomed to eating but with a twist in the carb content. The whole idea is to make a two week plan for what you will be eating during the induction phase. This way, there is no guessing. You know exactly what your meal strategy will be. Put this plan in writing. Draw up a diagram or list of what you will be eating for breakfast, snacks, lunch and dinner. Today, there are probably thousands of recipes on the web you can create and many are very simple. You do not need to be a chef. Many are just putting some ingredients together.

Speaking of ingredients, as soon as you have a plan in writing, go to the super market and buy these specific ingredients you will need. Be strong-willed and do not allow other family members to tempt you into buying processed foods that will just set you back on your diet plans. Cheating will only set you back. Make a strong commitment. When they see how you have slimmed down in such a short time, they will want to do the same and the whole family will follow your healthy diet for a healthier way of life for the whole family. The Atkins brand is now sold almost everywhere or you can save some money and do some yourself. The trick is to plan ahead. Stick to purchasing only the ingredients that you will need for your weekly diet plan. This will ensure success. It's simple.

Chapter 4: Developing the Right Eating Habits

Now, it's time to start making changes. The most important of which would be changing your eating habits and what you keep in your fridge. Stocking up before you start the diet can actually help you with following through and making sure that you don't end up skipping certain steps. To help you with this, here's a list of the different food items that you can enjoy during Phase 1 of the Atkins diet.

Produce (For Phase 1, you should be eating at least 15 grams of carbs per day in the form of veggies.)

Salads: Iceberg lettuce, Romaine lettuce, Spinach, Arugula and Endive.

Snacks: Celery, Cucumber and Peppers.

Salad Toppers: Avocados, Radishes, Mushrooms, Radicchio and Artichokes.

Side Dishes: Brussels sprouts, Snow Peas, Eggplant, Okra, Broccoli and Collard Greens.

Seasoning: Chives and Parsley.

Meat (All types of meat are allowed. The best ones are listed below.)

Fowl: Cornish Hen, Chicken, Duck and Turkey.

Meat: Beef, Bacon, Lamb, Ham and Pork.

Seafood (All types of shellfish and fish are allowed.)

Fish: Halibut, Salmon, Cod, Tuna and Trout.

Shellfish: Shrimp, Clams, Oysters, Crabmeat and Mussels.

Dairy: Mayonnaise and Sour Cream.

Cheeses: Goat Cheese, Swiss, Blue, Parmesan, Cheddar, Feta, Mozzarella, Cream Cheese, Gouda and American cheese.

Staples: Lemon juice, Lime juice, Eggs, Salad dressing, Vegetable oil, Splenda, Olive oil, Bouillon cubes, Vegetable or chicken broth and spices for flavoring.

Beverages: Club soda, Zero calorie seltzer water, Tea, Diet Soda, Coffee and Club soda.

Things to Keep In Mind:

- You will go through an adjustment period once you start with the Atkins diet. You might find that during the first few days, your energy is a little lower than usual. However, this should change after a few more days. In fact, most people tend to feel lighter and far less lethargic once the first week is over.

- Because of the change in your diet, you will experience weight loss. This might seem sudden to some but don't fret! Remember that this is simply water weight.

- Always make sure that you're drinking 8 glasses of water each day. This is vital to both your health and progress when it comes to losing weight. Water is essential when it comes to metabolizing any stored fat and as such, if you're constantly dehydrated, your metabolism won't be as active. Cold water is best for this purpose.

- Make sure that you read the labels for every food item you buy. Doing so would allow you to get familiar with carb counts. Another thing you can do is get a carb counter and keep it with you all the time. Having it handy should help you quickly decide if a certain type of food fits within your allotted carb total for the day.

- Reduce your coffee intake. This would help you lose weight faster because drinking too much of it can lead to insulin increase in your body—this would then hinder the speed at which your body burns away fat.

- Feeling weaker than usual? This might mean that you're not getting the sufficient amount of carbs needed. Keep in mind that the Atkins diet is LOW CARBS not NO CARBS. Try adding a bit more to your daily meals and see if that changes anything. It's all about finding the right balance for yourself as this can vary from one person to the next.

Chapter 5: Common Atkins Diet Mistakes to Avoid

As with anything that you're trying out for the first time, mistakes are almost inevitable. However, when it comes to the Atkin's diet, this shouldn't be the case. There are certain issues that can be avoided easily if one were to simply take the time when it comes to learning more about the diet. To help you out, here are 3 of the most common mistakes that people do during the diet, as well as the different ways they can be avoided.

- Counting total carbs and discounting net carbs.

When on the Atkin's diet, remember that you need to count the net carbs which is basically the total grams of carbs in your food minus that of fiber's—the latter has no effect whatsoever on your blood sugar after all. Another thing to remember is to count the carb content of condiments as well as lemon juice. Try not to use all of your daily carb allowance on foods that are also high in sugar starch but low in fiber content. To better understand this, a carb chart and a carb counter would be helpful.

- Not eating enough protein.

As a general rule, you should eat 4 to 6 ounces of protein with every meal. This can change depending on your height and gender, however. 4 ounces is usually enough for petite women whilst a man might need around 6 ounces. What happens if you skimp on protein? Well, this could greatly affect your weight loss and can leave you feeling hungry all the time. You might find that your carb cravings have resurfaced and you're more prone to breaking the cycle or quitting the diet completely. To avoid this, always make sure that you're getting the right amount for yourself. Remember, the same applies to having too much of it in your diet.

- Being afraid of fat and calories.

This is one of the primary mistakes that beginners make. Always remember that dietary fat is essential to help stimulate the body's ability to burn it. Having more natural fats in your diet is completely okay as long as you control your carb intake to balance it out. If you're having a snack that contains some carbs, always balance it out with fat or protein. For example, if you're having cucumber slices then do make sure you take it with some cheese—or even bacon bits. When it comes to this, moderation and balance is the key. Keep in mind that too much of one thing can become bad for your health as well.

Remember that there are good fats and bad fats so make sure that you choose your source well. Keep it natural and organic as much as possible.

Chapter 6: Eating Out While on the Atkins Diet

Love eating out? Of course you do – almost everyone does. However, heading out to your favorite restaurant for dinner can have some dire consequences if you aren't careful. Luckily, there are a few things that you can do to ensure you stick to your Atkins Diet and still enjoy going out to eat every once in a while.

Whether your favorite food is Chinese, Mexican or Italian, as long as you stick to a few small guidelines, you can eat out without feeling guilty! Keep reading to find out these guidelines, as well as a few tips to help you along the way, and some great food items that are on some of your favorite fast food restaurant menus. I'll even help you determine low-carb eating solutions for Chinese, Italian and Mexican restaurants.

Eating Out at Mexican Restaurants

While there are plenty of items to avoid at a Mexican restaurant, there's also plenty that is safe for you. You'll want to skip the chips and salsa; although, I know, they look so appetizing. You can, however, have the guacamole with your entrée. Speaking of your entrée, you'll want to stick to a few items, such as grilled meats and seafood. You can have fajitas and tostado salads, but skill the tortillas and shell. If you want to opt for a stew/soup dish, have the chili verde.

Ultimately, at a Mexican restaurant, here's what you want to avoid: tacos, tortillas, burritos, nachos, taquitos, enchiladas, quesadillas, tamales, flautas, and chimichangas. The reason these are on the avoid list is because of the outside shell, so if you want to order just the filling of a chimichanga, go right ahead.

Eating Out at McDonald's

As the largest fast food chain worldwide, McDonald's is a hard habit to break when you go on a diet. When ordering a burger from McDonald's, you will want to order it without the bun – or take the bun off when you get it. This removes the carbs. The cheese and vegetables will have about one gram of carbohydrates each and Big Mac sauce and ketchup will have about two grams.

If you opt for chicken or fish, be careful because you will get a decent amount of carbs, depending on how it's cooked. For example, grilled chicken only has a couple of grams of carbs while the Filet-o-Fish and crispy chicken has 9-10 grams of carbs each.

If you opt for salad, you'll only get about three grams of carbs with the side salad – and plenty of nutrition and greens! Salad with grilled chicken nets about 9 grams of carbs and crispy chicken salads have as much as 38 carbs. Stick to Caesar Salads and Bacon Ranch Salads with GRILLED chicken to limit your carb intake.

Don't even think about eating McNuggets, French fries or any type of dessert from McDonald's. You'll totally botch your diet if you do.

For eating at McDonald's, try this tool: **http://www.mcdonalds.com/us/en/food.html**. It is a tool that is obviously available on the McDonald's website. It allows you to view any item on their menu and click/un-click certain parts of that item, such as the bun, to see the amount of carbs.

Eating Out at Burger King

The same advice goes for Burger King as it did for McDonald's. Eat without the bun. Opt for grilled chicken sandwiches, as they'll only have a few grams of carbs. In fact, the only sensible low-carb Atkins-approved chicken sandwich at Burger King is the Tendergrill Chicken Sandwich with 3 grams of carbs – without the bun. The Tendergrill is the only logical salad choice, as well, at 8 grams.

Eating Out at Subway

Obviously, Subway is healthier than McDonald's and Burger King, but do they have anything for low-carb, Atkins Diet followers? Unfortunately, because the tortillas and bread have so many carbs, there are not many options at Subway when on the Atkins Diet. You are going to have to opt for salads, netting about 10 grams of carbs. Choose your dressing wisely though – the oil and vinegar has zero carbs while the red wine vinaigrette has about 17 carbs.

Eating Out at Chinese Restaurants

When eating out at a Chinese restaurant, you must be careful or you'll quickly consume too many carbs. You will want to avoid rice, noodles, wontons, egg rolls and breaded meats. Your best bets are going to be stir-fried dishes, steamed foods, clear and thin soups and walnut chicken. If you choose a meat and vegetable combination or any other dish, limit the sauce, especially if it is thick and spicy, as this means more starch and sugar. If you aren't careful, you could take in about seven grams of carbohydrates with just one tablespoon of cornstarch. If all else fails, ask for the sauce to be on the side.

Eating Out at Italian Restaurants

Sure, Italian food consists of pizza, pasta and delicious bread –
all of which are full of carbohydrates – but that doesn't mean
that there aren't some decent, low-carb dishes that you can
savor while on the Atkins Diet. When it comes to appetizers,
stick to seafood, meats and veggies.

If you want soup, you'll want to stick to the thinner soups, such
as seafood soups, Stracciatelle and vegetable soups. Obviously,
a salad is a fine choice while on Atkins, but avoid the croutons.
The variety of seafood and meats on the menu will be fine, as
long as you steer clear of the breaded meats.

General Eating Out Tips

Before we just delve into foods that you can eat when dining
out, let's look at a few basic principles.

1.   Order foods with plenty of protein and fiber.

2.   Avoid trans fat.

3.   Choose leafy greens.

4.   Avoid refined sugars.

5.   Opt for grilled chicken instead of crispy chicken.

6.   Always do away with the bun/bread on burgers and
sandwiches.

7.   Don't be afraid to take your own spices/dressing to the
restaurant.

8.   Always start your meal with a healthy salad. (Low carbs,
high fiber)

9.   Ask for substitutions. Usually, to keep your service,
restaurants will accommodate your request.

Chapter 7: How to Accelerate Weight Loss

It's great that you've decided to try the Atkins Diet to lose weight, but you honestly need to do more than just diet. While you will lose weight dieting alone, you could increase the amount of weight that you lose and speed up the pounds shedding off if you add an exercise regimen into your weight loss program.

The best way to reach your goal weight is to make lifestyle changes, which includes the Atkins Diet and sweating it out at the gym or at home on a regular basis. Here are some tips to help you speed up the weight loss process and simply stay on top of things:

1.   **Use your scale.** Don't weight yourself every single day. Instead, only weigh in about once per week. Try to make it on the same day and at the same time. The best time to weigh yourself is first thing in the morning before you have put anything in your body and your digestive system is clean.

2.   **Exercise regularly.** To speed up weight loss now and to keep the weight off in the future, it's important to exercise. You should perform around 2-3 hours per week of moderate intensity aerobic exercise or half of that of vigorous intensity. In addition, you should spend two days or more focusing on strength training each muscle group.

3.   **Make sure you have plenty of support around you.** It can be hard to stick to a diet and exercise activity if you don't have support of family and friends. In some cases, many dieters find that support will actually help speed up the weight loss process because they stay on track.

4.   **Fight your food cravings.** Giving into your food cravings is a definite way to slow down the process of losing weight. Not only will you eat more than you should, but you will also start gaining your weight back. You will want to make sure that when you start on the Atkins Diet that you remove all prohibited foods from your home (soda, candy, ice cream, etc.). Fill your home with the healthy, low-carb foods that you can have.

5.   **Do not starve yourself.** This is the quickest way to hurt yourself and to do damage to your dieting efforts. You aren't going to be doing your body any good starving it. Did you know that when you skip meals it can actually cause you to have excessive hunger pains? We all know hunger pains only lead to trouble!

6.   **Beware of binge eating.** When you get stressed out or have a lot on your plate, it is possible that you will begin to binge eat, which is when you eat a large amount of food without a short period of time. This will most definitely harm your weight loss process. Instead of perusing the fridge for carbs, head out for a brisk walk or go to the gym to get your mind on something else.

7.   **Consider a diet buddy.** Sometimes it can be heard to diet and exercise alone. If you have someone that wants to lose weight as much as you, then it can actually be fun to exercise. You can share motivational tips and recipes while keeping each other on track.

Remember, you are responsible for your weight loss. No one and nothing else. If you can't put in the time and effort to shed those unwanted pounds, then you aren't going to get that slim, sexy body that you've always dreamed of. Set yourself some goals and stick to your diet and exercise regimen. It's the only way to lose weight.

Chapter 8: How to Keep the Weight Off

Did you know that probably about 90 percent of all dieters that lose weight while on a diet regain that weight or at least a portion of that weight within a year's time? You don't want to be in that 90 percent.

Aside from sticking to the maintenance phase of the Atkins Diet, there are plenty of other ways that you can help yourself keep the weight off. Here are some tips on how to keep the weight off:

☐ Exercise on a daily basis or at least as often as possible. Use every opportunity you have to exercise, even if it's just 15 minutes.

☐ Make sure resistance training is part of your exercise workout. This will help you maintain muscle mass.

☐ Don't start stuffing your face with carbs. You've worked so hard to get to where you are, and you did that by eating fewer carbs each day. Don't damage everything you've done so far by getting addicted to carbs again.

☐ Reduce fried and refined foods, as these are empty calories.

☐ Stay hydrated. Water ensures that your metabolism is strong and continues to burn calories efficiently.

☐ Keep your stress levels as stable as possible. When you become stressed, cortisol is produced raising insulin resistance and encouraging storage of fat.

☐	Make sure to get as much sleep as possible. Adults need about eight hours of sleep per night.

☐	Continue to weigh yourself on a regular basis so that if you do start to gain weight, you catch it early on and can get those pounds off quickly.

Exercise is most definitely going to be one of the best ways to keep the weight off after you lose it. There are various programs out there, such as Zumba and CrossFit, so that you don't just head out to the gym and get on a boring treadmill. If you are looking for a great guide to CrossFit, I would highly recommend you check out this guide; ***CrossFit: Ultimate Guide to CrossFit Training and Feeling Amazing!*** Exercise can become tedious after a while if you don't shake things up a bit. Taking a dance class or swimming a few laps around the pool can help keep things fresh so that you aren't always at the gym working out. Also, try amping up your workouts. If you've been walking for 30 minutes, try adding another 30 minutes to that or turning your walk into a jog.

You've lost the weight and now all you have to do is keep it off. If you continue eating healthy and exercising regularly, you'll find that it's quite easy to keep the weight off and maintain a tone body.

Chapter 9: Breakfast Recipes

Ham Rollups

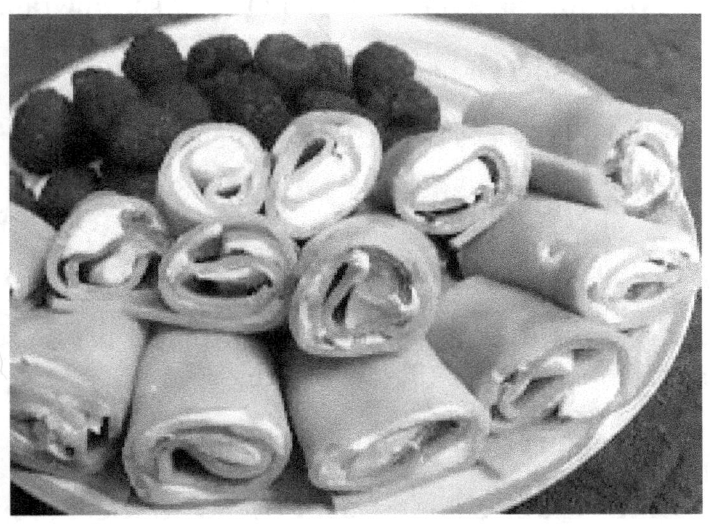

Prep time: 9 minutes

Cook time: 0 minutes

Serves: 6

Ingredients

- 6 Tortilla Factory low carb whole wheat tortillas

- 8 oz. whipped cream cheese

- 6 slices ham, the rectangular kind, cut in half

- ½ cup pickle dill relish

- 2 tablespoon mayonnaise

- 2 tablespoon Dijon mustard

Directions

1. Combine cream cheese, dill relish, mustard and mayo in a bowl.

2. Lay one tortilla out on waxed paper or saran wrap.

3. Place one slice of ham on top.

4. Spread ham slices with the cream cheese mixture.

5. Roll the entire piece up.

6. Cut in half.

7. Refrigerate until serving, 1 whole tortilla is one serving, so if cut in half, is still one serving.

8. Place serving size per individual zip-lock bag.

Nutritional Value: Calories: 228, Total Fat: 18g, Protein: 18g, Total Carbs: 6g, Dietary Fiber: 7g, Sugar: 0g, Sodium: 358mg

Junior Mint Shake

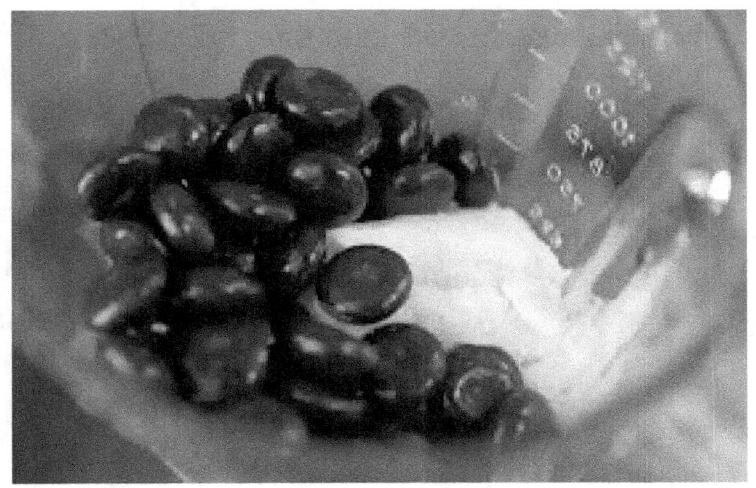

Prep time: 4 minutes

Cook time: 0

Serves: 1

Ingredients

- 2 tablespoon cocoa

- 6 oz. COLD water

- ¼ cup protein powder or chocolate

- 3 drops peppermint flavoring

- ½ cup cottage cheese

- 2 packets sweetener

- 5 ice cubes

Directions

1. Mix the ingredients and emulsify by blending.

2. Blend until thick.

3. Combine dry ingredients and place in zip-lock bag. Combine cottage cheese and sweetener and refrigerate.

Nutritional Value: Calories: 200, Total Fat: 2g, Protein: 39g, Total Carbs: 7g, Dietary Fiber: 1g, Sugar: 3g, Sodium: 348mg

Sausage Egg Muffins

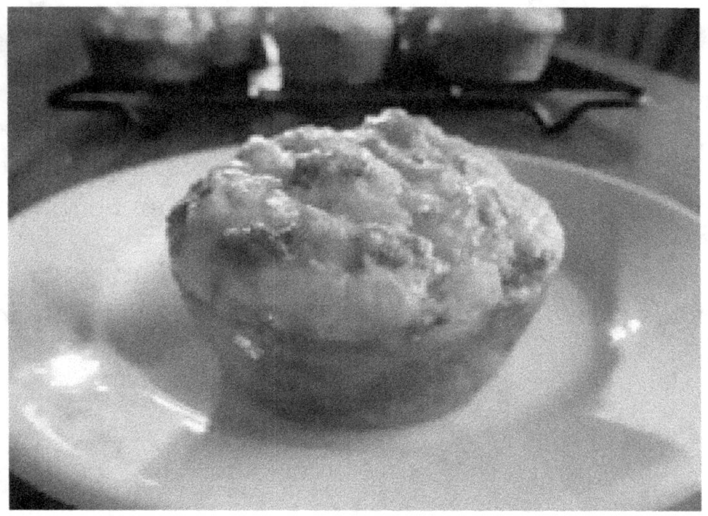

Prep time: 10minutes

Cook time: 29 minutes

Serves: 12

Ingredients

- 12 oz. cooked sausage crumbles

- 12 eggs

- ¼ cup milk

- 2 cups cheddar cheese, sharp, hand-shredded

- ¼ tablespoon black pepper or chili pepper

Directions

1. Mix all the ingredients.

2. Pour into 12 greased muffin papers (in a pan).

3. Bake at 375 degrees for 29 minutes.

4. Cool for 4 minutes before serving.

Freezing Instructions

5. After cooling, place in zip-lock freezer bag. For the best
    flavor, heat in microwave or toaster oven before eating.

Nutritional Value: Calories: 200, Total Fat: 39g, Protein:
16g, Total Carbs: 2g, Dietary Fiber: 0g, Sugar: 0, Sodium:
370mg

Chocolate Muffin

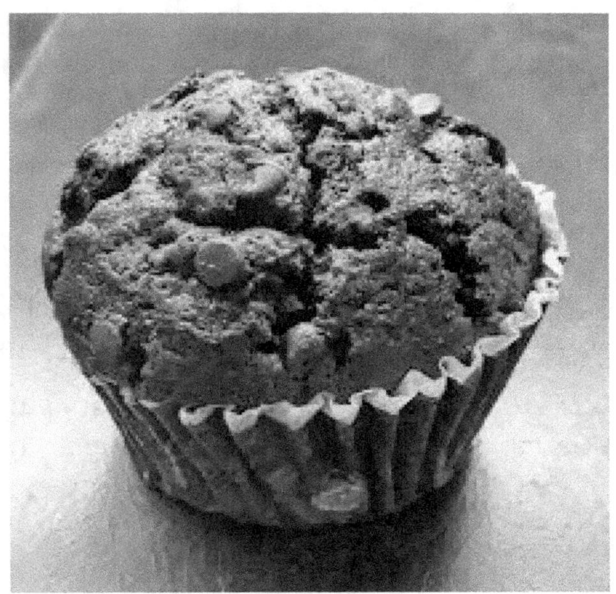

Prep time: 4 minutes

Cook time: 1 minutes

Serves: 1

Ingredients

- 1 tablespoon plain flour

- 1 scoop of Chocolate Protein Powder

- ½ tablespoon baking powder

- 1 tablespoon of cocoa powder

- 2 packets Splenda

- 1 tablespoon butter

- 1 egg

Directions

1. Mix the dry ingredients in a cup

2. Combine the wet ingredients

3. Add the wet ingredients into the cup of dry

4. Microwave for one minute

5. Place individual muffins in a zip-lock bag and place in the freezer. Microwave one minute to thaw and serve.

Nutritional Value: Calories: 207, Total Fat: 24g, Protein: 10g, Total Carbs: 16, Dietary Fiber: 11g, Sugar: 0, Sodium: 308mg

Spicy Deviled Eggs

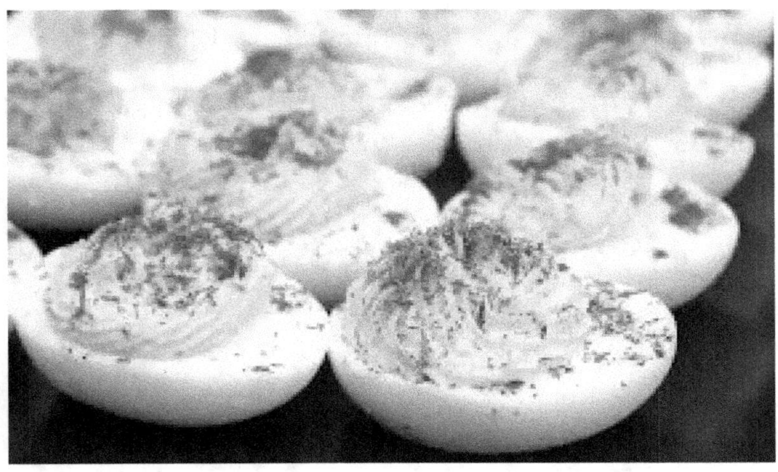

Prep time: 9 minutes

Cook time: 11 minutes

Serves: 2

Ingredients

- 4 hard-boiled eggs

- 2 tablespoon mayonnaise

- 1 tablespoon spicy brown mustard

- 1 tablespoon diced green chilies

Directions

1. Boil the eggs for 9 minutes.

2. Slice the eggs in half.

3. Scoop out the yolks.

4. Mix the yolks, the mayo, the mustard and the chilies.

5. Place back in the center of the egg whites.

6. Boil the eggs in advance and place in the fridge.

Nutritional Value: Calories: 202, Total Fat: 15g, Protein: 12g, Total Carbs: 3, Dietary Fiber: 0g, Sugar: 2g, Sodium: 20mg

Butter Pecan Waffles

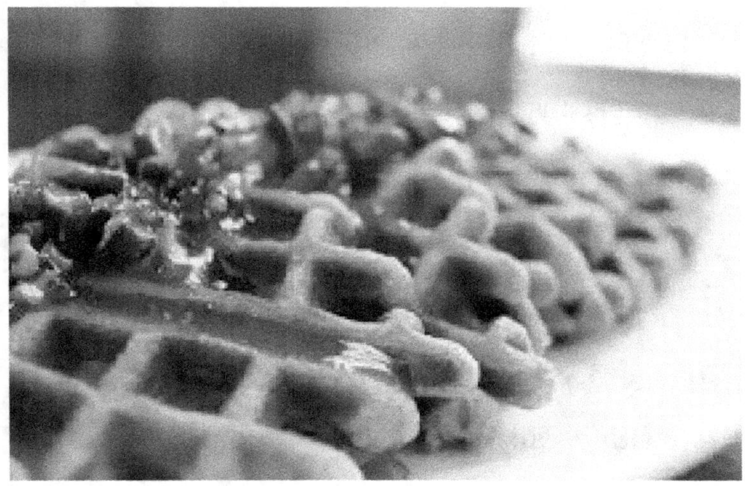

Prep time: 9 minutes

Cook time: 4 minutes

Serves: 8

Ingredients

- 1 cup soy flour

- 2 packets Splenda

- 3 tablespoon baking powder

- ¾ cup buttermilk

- 1 tablespoon butter

- ½ tablespoon baking soda

- 3 eggs

- 2 tablespoon vanilla

- ½ cup water

- 2 tablespoon sugar free butter rum flavoring

- ½ cup pecans

Directions

1. Combine everything except the pecans.

2. Use ¼ c batter for cooking the waffle.

3. Cook until crisp.

4. Top with pecans and sugar free syrup.

5. After the waffle is cool, place 1 per zip-lock bag. Warm by toasting in the toaster.

Nutritional Value: Calories: 181, Total Fat: 13g, Protein: 9g, Total Carbs: 5g, Dietary Fiber: 2g, Sugar: 3g, Sodium: 178mg

Huevos Rancheros

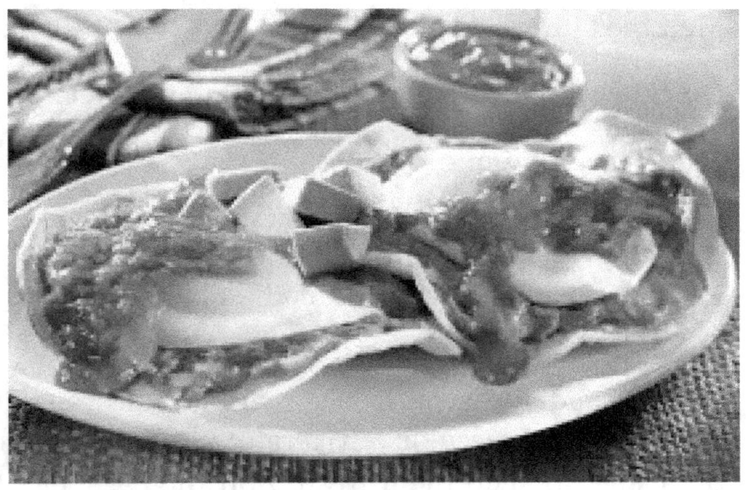

Prep time: 9 minutes

Cook time: 19 minutes

Serves: 4

Ingredients

- 4 oz. cooked ground sirloin

- ½ cup Pace Salsa Verde

- 4 eggs

- 4 slices Canadian bacon

- 4 Tortilla Factory Low Carb Whole Wheat tortillas

- 4 tablespoon water

- 4 tablespoon butter

Directions

1. Melt the butter in a glass bowl.

2. Quickly whip the egg and water with the butter.

3. Microwave 1 minute.

4. Place the tortilla in the microwave for 10 seconds.

5. Layer as follows: Tortilla, Canadian bacon, ground beef, egg, salsa.

6. Place Canadian bacon, cooked sirloin, and salsa into a zip-lock bag. Freeze or refrigerate. Place the tortillas in the fridge to keep them fresh. Add the eggs, etc. when microwaving

Nutritional Value: Calories: 277, Total Fat: 17g, Protein: 20g, Total Carbs: 8g, Dietary Fiber: 13g, Sugar: 3g, Sodium: 720mg

Denver Omelet

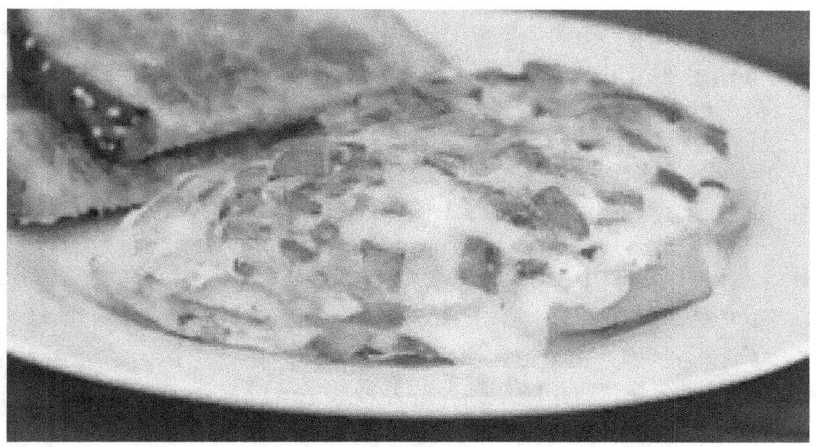

Prep time: 4 minutes

Cook time: 1 minutes

Serves: 1

Ingredients

- 2 tablespoon butter
- ¼ cup chopped onions
- ¼ cup green bell pepper, diced
- ¼ cup halved grape tomatoes
- 2 eggs
- ¼ cup chopped ham

Directions

1. Sautee the onions and bell pepper, with the butter, in a small skillet.

2. Whip the eggs and mix the ingredients in a bowl.

3. Microwave for one minute.

4. Pre-cook the peppers and onions and place in zip-lock freezer bags by portions, add the ham to the bags. Freeze. The night before making, place the peppers mix in the fridge to thaw or microwave for one minute before adding to the whipped egg to make.

Nutritional Value: Calories: 605, Total Fat: 46g, Protein: 39g, Total Carbs: 6g, Dietary Fiber: 2g, Sugar: 0g, Sodium: 380mg

Breakfast Mexican Omelet

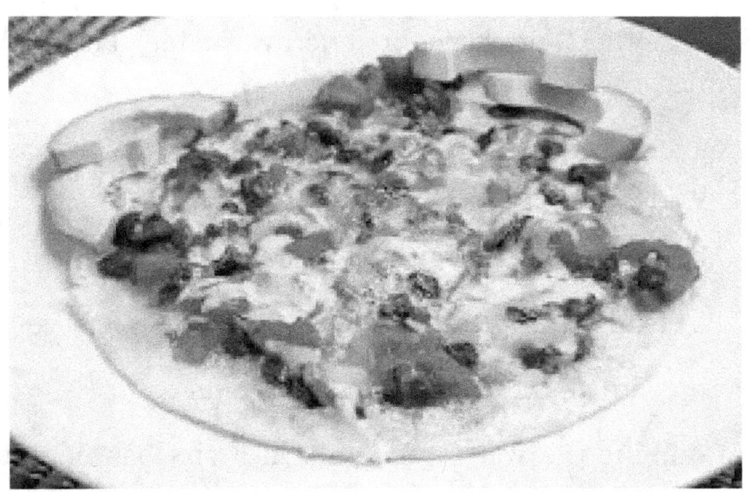

Prep time: 4 minutes

Cook time: 9 minutes

Serves: 1

Ingredients

- ½ tablespoon lime juice

- 2 eggs 1 tablespoon water

- 1 tablespoon crumbled bacon

- 1/2 tablespoon butter

- ¼ avocado

- ½ cup hand-shredded Mexican cheese

- 2 tablespoon Pace Thick and Chunky Medium Salsa

Directions

1. Melt the butter in a microwaveable bowl in the microwave.

2. Quickly whip the wet ingredients in a microwaveable bowl, can be the same bowl as before.

3. Microwave for one minute.

4. Place on warm plate.

5. Top with all the rest of the ingredients.

6. Combine the wet ingredients in a zip-lock bag, except the butter and water. Refrigerate. Combine the water and butter in a zip-lock bag.

Nutritional Value: Calories: 275, Total Fat: 21, Protein: 17g, Total Carbs: 3.2g, Dietary Fiber: 2g, Sugar: 2g, Sodium: 230mg

Cinnamon Chocolate Smoothie

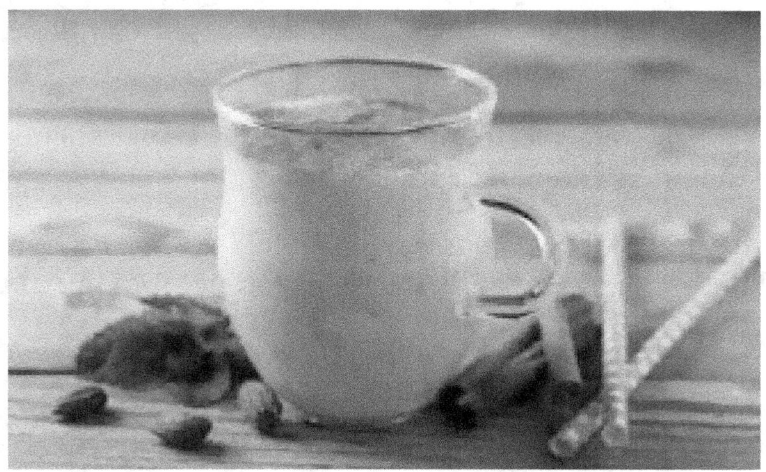

Prep time: 4 minutes

Cook time: 0 minutes

Serves: 1

Ingredients

- ½ cup firm Tofu

- 2 tablespoon cocoa powder

- 1 scoop chocolate protein powder

- 2 tablespoon cinnamon

- 2 sweetener packets

- 1 cup almond milk, unsweetened

- 4 ice cubes

Directions

1. Place all the ingredients in a blender, pulse until desired consistency, and serve.

2. Refrigerate the tofu. Place all the dry ingredients into one snack sized zip-lock bag.

Nutritional Value: Calories: 273, Total Fat: 15g, Protein: 33g, Total Carbs: 9g, Dietary Fiber: 20g, Sugar: 2g, Sodium: 214mg

Cheese Blintz with Blueberries

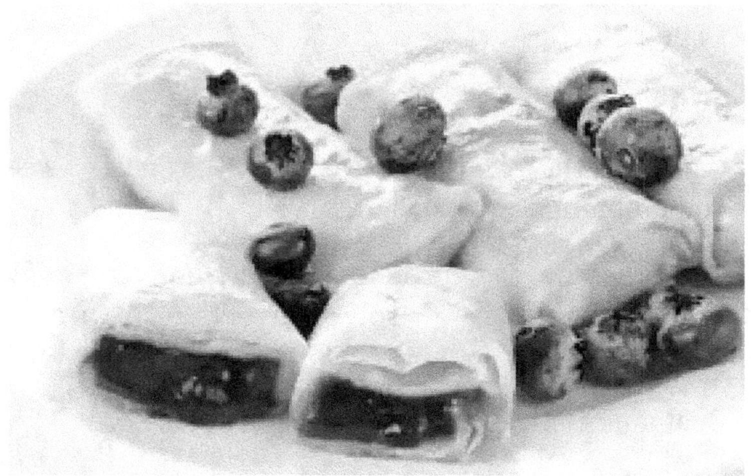

Prep time: 9 minutes

Cook time: 4 minutes

Serves: 1

Ingredients

- 1 medium egg

- 1 tablespoon half & half

- 1 scoop protein shake powder, vanilla

- 1 pat of butter

- 1 tablespoon of olive oil

- 2 tablespoon ricotta cheese

- 1 tablespoon Greek yogurt, plain

- 1 packet sweetener

- 1 tablespoon cinnamon

- ½ cup blueberries

Directions

1. Combine the ricotta cheese, Greek yogurt, sweetener and cinnamon in a bowl, mix well.

2. Combine the egg, protein powder, and cream. Whisk until all lumps are dissolved, and the mixture is well-blended.

3. Coat a non-stick skillet with the olive oil.

4. At medium heat, melt butter in the skillet and pour the batter on top.

5. Swirl the skillet until the batter is evenly distributed. When the batter has set, gently turn the blintz to the other side.

6. Let cook for one minute until the batter is set, but not browned.

7. Gently fold half the blueberries into the filling.

8. Place the filling in the middle of the blitz.

9. Roll into a pancake and serve with the remaining blueberries.

10. Mix the filling and place in the fridge in a covered container. Place the blueberries in a zip-lock bag and place in the freezer.

Nutritional Value: Calories: 427 Total Fat: 23g, Protein: 39g, Total Carbs: 14g, Dietary Fiber: 3g, Sugar: 10g, Sodium: 330mg

Spinach and Swiss Quiche

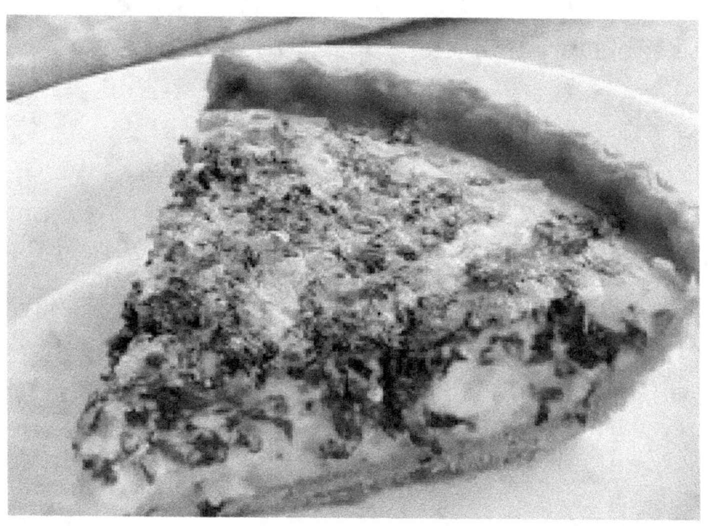

Prep time: 19 minutes

Cook time: 29 minutes

Serves: 4

Ingredients

- 2 tablespoon butter

- 6 oz. frozen chopped spinach, drained and thawed

- 1 cup cream

- 1 cup hand-shredded swiss cheese or hand-shredded cheese

- ¼ tablespoon salt

- 1 diced white onion

- 4 eggs

- ⅛ tablespoon nutmeg

- ¼ tablespoon black pepper, ground

Directions

1. Heat the oven to 350 degrees.

2. Then spray a pie pan with your choice of cooking spray. Spray liberally as eggs may stick.

3. Cook onions in butter till glassy, then add the spinach and simmer until the water is gone.

4. Mix all of the ingredients in a bowl, including the spices.

5. Pour into the pie pan.

6. Bake for 29 minutes.

7. Cool for 9 minutes and cut into quarters.

8. Wrap a cooled slice of quiche in saran wrap, then place in a zip-lock bag. Microwave for 1 minute in two 30-second bursts.

Nutritional Value: Calories: 417, Total Fat: 37g, Protein: 15g, Total Carbs: 4g, Dietary Fiber: 1.5g, Sugar: 0g, Sodium: 209mg

Chapter 10: Lunch

Cobb Salad

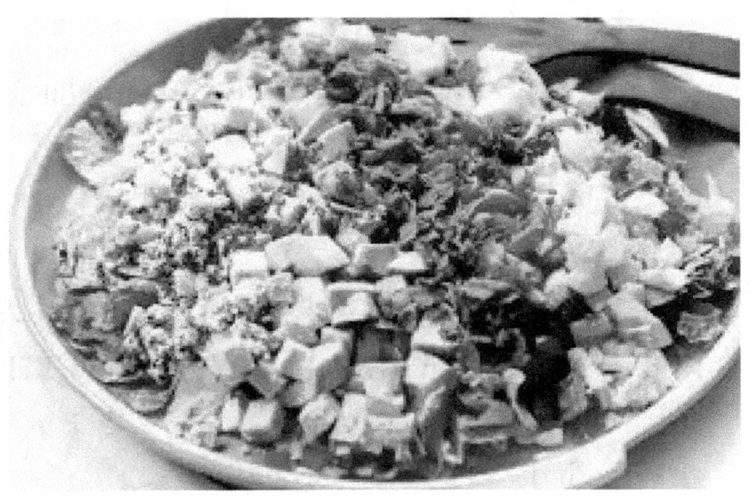

Prep time: 9 minutes

Cook time: 9 minutes

Serves: 1

Ingredients

- 1 slice Bacon or 1 tablespoon real bacon bits

- 1 grilled Chicken Breast, which has been cut into thin strips

- 1 cup Spring Mix Salad

- 1/2 cup grape tomatoes, sliced in half

- ½ avocado, sliced into small moons

- ¼ cup pepper jack cheese, hand-shredded

- 2 tablespoon Ken's Buttermilk Ranch Dressing

Directions

1. Assemble ingredients by sections.

2. Cover the entire bottom of the plate with lettuce.

3. In one corner (relative if you have a round plate) place the tomatoes.

4. In the opposite section place the avocado strips in a fan shape.

5. In the third section place the bacon bits.

6. In the fourth section place the hand-shredded cheese. In the center place the chicken.

7. Drizzle with the salad dressing and serve.

8. The chicken can be frozen in a zip-lock bag. Microwave 1 minute to serve. The salad can be combined in one bowl or packed in individual containers and placed in the fridge.

Nutritional Value: Calories: 561, Total Fat: 34g, Protein: 51g, Total Carbs: 3.9g, Dietary Fiber: 6g, Sugar: 1g, Sodium: 802mg

Shrimp and Cucumber Salad

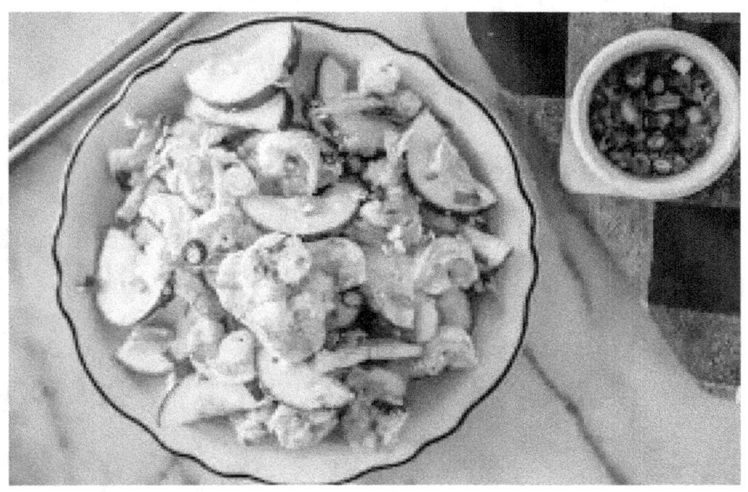

Prep time: 4 minutes

Cook time: 0 minutes

Serves: 4

Ingredients

- 2 English cucumbers

- 1/4 cup of red wine vinegar

- 2 tablespoon of Splenda

- 1/4 tablespoon salt

- ½ cup cooked shrimp

Directions

1. Peel the cucumbers so that they have stripes down the side.

2. Slice the cucumbers as thin as you can.

3. Mix the dressing of sugar, salt, and vinegar very well

4. Place the cucumbers on a plate

5. Place the shrimp on top

6. Add the dressing and serve.

7. Create the entire salad and place in a covered container in the fridge. Will keep 2 days.

Nutritional Value: Calories: 26g, Total Fat: 0g, Protein: 2g, Total Carbs: 3g, Dietary Fiber: 2g, Sugar: 2g, Sodium: 157mg

Feta Cucumber Salad

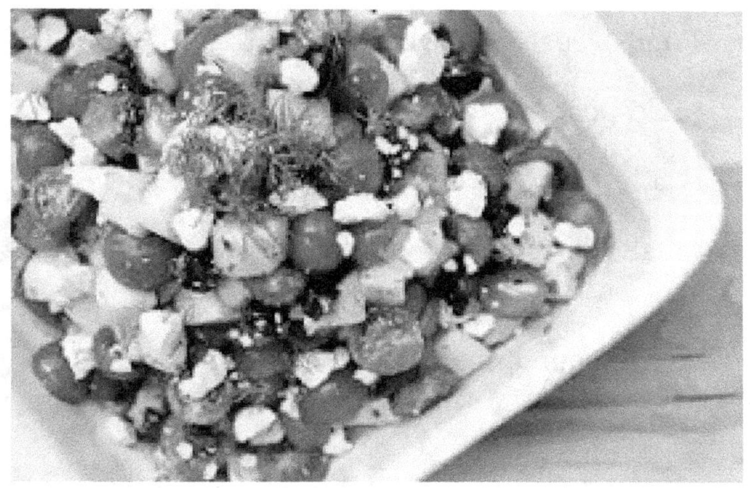

Prep time: 14 minutes

Cook time: none

Serves: 4

Ingredients

- 1 head of leaf lettuce, coarsely chopped

- 1 cup baby spinach, trimmed, coarsely chopped

- ½ cup diced red onion

- 1 cup grape tomatoes, sliced in half

- ¼ cup Feta cheese, crumbled

- 2 cups plain greek yogurt

- 2 tablespoon garlic powder

- 1 tablespoon dill

- 2 tablespoon lemon juice

- 2 English cucumbers, chopped with peels on

- 2 tablespoon olive oil

- ¼ tablespoon black pepper

- 1 small can black olives, sliced and drained (2.25 oz. can)

- ½ tablespoon mint or 3 mint leaves

Directions

1. Combine Greek yogurt, dill, garlic powder, mint, lemon juice, olive oil, ½ cup diced cucumber, and black pepper and emulsify by blending.

2. Taste and add salt. Add water by tablespoons if too thick.

3. Arrange on 4 plates the lettuce and spinach, tomatoes, cucumbers, and black olives.

4. Pour the dressing over the salad.

5. Top with the feta cheese.

6. Mix the salad dressing and place in fridge in closed containers. Mix the salad and bag or place in covered containers in the fridge.

7. Place the feta cheese in a zip-lock bag in the fridge.

Nutritional Value: Calories: 142, Total Fat: 10g, Protein: 4g, Total Carbs: 7g, Dietary Fiber: 3g, Sugar: 0g, Sodium: 144mg

Stuffed with goat cheese,

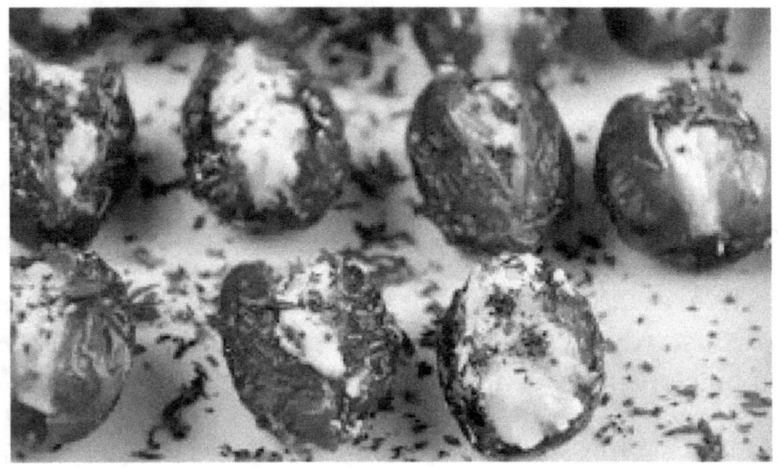

Prep Time: 5 Hours and 30 Minutes

Serves: 4

Ingredients:

- ¼ cup of red wine

- ¼ cup of balsamic vinegar

- 2 tablespoon of Dijon mustard

- 2 tablespoon of soy sauce

- 1 cup of extra virgin olive oil

- 4 cloves of garlic, peeled and thinly sliced

- 1 tablespoon of salt Dash of black pepper

- 1, 2 to 3 pounds of flank steak

Ingredients for the stuffing:

- ½ cup of pancetta, cooked and chopped

- 8 ounces of goat cheese

- 3 cups of spinach, drained and excess liquid drained

Directions:

1. Use a large bowl and add in the red wine, vinegar, mustard, soy sauce, olive oil, garlic and dash of salt and black pepper. Whisk until mixed.

2. Add in the flank steak and cover. Set in the fridge to marinate for 4 hours.

3. Place a large saucepan over low heat. Chop the pancetta and place into the saucepan. Cook for 20 to 30 minutes. Drain the excess fat and set the pancetta aside.

4. Add the spinach into the saucepan and cook for 1 to 2 minutes or until fragrant. Remove from the pan and squeeze out the excess liquid. Add into a bowl with the pancetta and goat cheese. Stir well to mix.

5. Remove the flank steak from the marinade and place onto a flat surface. Beat with a meat mallet until ¼ inch in thickness.

6. Spread the stuffing onto the flank steak. Roll and tie with twine to seal. Season with a dash of salt and black pepper.

7. Heat up the oven to 400 degrees.

8. Place the rolled flank steak onto a large baking sheet and drizzle a few drops of olive oil over the top.

9. Place into the oven to bake for 15 to 25 minutes or until cooked through. Remove and allow to rest for 15 minutes before serving.

Nutritional Value: Calories: 646, Fat: 58 grams, Carbs: 4 grams, Protein: 27 grams

Chicken Lettuce Wraps

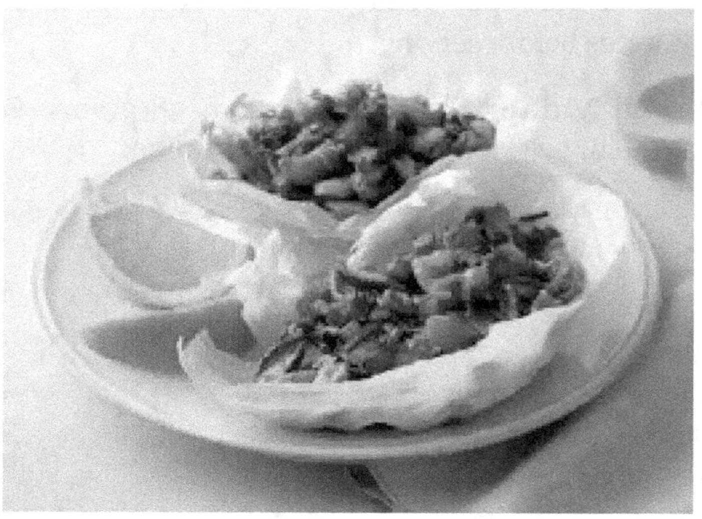

Prep time: 10minutes

Cook time: 10minutes

Serves: 1

Ingredients

- 1 chicken breast, boneless, diced into 1-inch size pieces

- 1 cup diced or sliced fresh mushrooms

- ½ cup diced water chestnuts (from a can, drained)

- 1 tablespoon olive oil

- 1 tablespoon onion, minced

- 1 tablespoon minced garlic

- 1 tablespoon teriyaki sauce

- garlic powder, only a dash

- onion powder, just a dash

- oregano, one dash

- cayenne pepper, a small dash

- salt /pepper

Directions

1. Mix the ingredients and cook in a skillet until the chicken is done, about 10 minutes.

2. Shred the chicken

3. Place in leaves and roll

4. Place all ingredients into one freezer bag except the lettuce. Microwave one minute and serve.

Nutritional Value: Calories: 145, Total Fat: 1g, Protein: 35g, Dietary Fiber: 1g, Total Carbs: 4g, Sugar: 0g, Sodium: 100mg

Chicken Quesadillas

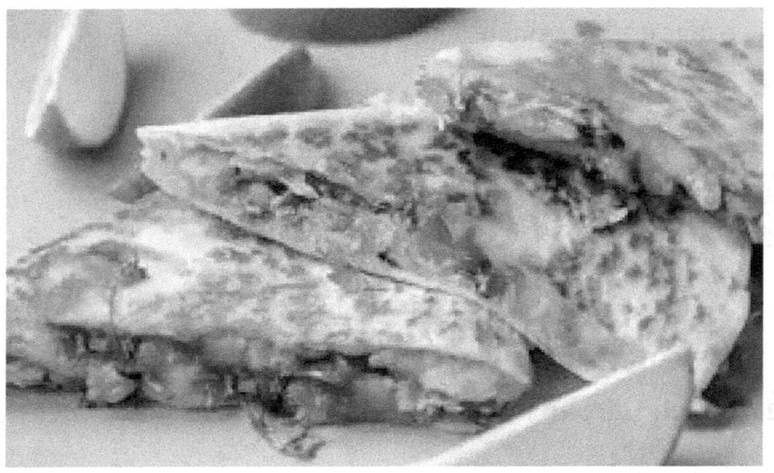

Prep time: 4 minutes

Cook time: 4 minutes

Serves: 4

Ingredients

- 1 cup pepper jack cheese, hand-shredded

- 8 tortillas Tortilla Factory Low Carb Whole Wheat Tortillas

- 8 oz. cooked and shredded Chicken Breast

- 1 chopped and Roasted Bell Pepper

- 2 tablespoon Cilantro

- 2 tablespoon Butter

- 1 cup plain Greek yogurt

Directions

1. Place ½ pat of butter in a skillet

2. Mix all the ingredients in a bowl except the yogurt

3. Place meat ingredients inside tortillas

4. Toast each side

5. Cut into 4 wedges

6. Top with yogurt and salsa, if desired

7. Freeze in zip-lock bags. Place the yogurt in the fridge. Heat one minute in the microwave to thaw.

Nutritional Value: Calories: 425g, Total Fat: 25g, Protein: 44g, Total Carbs: 10g, Dietary Fiber: 9g, Sugar: 2g, Sodium: 186mg

Chili Mac

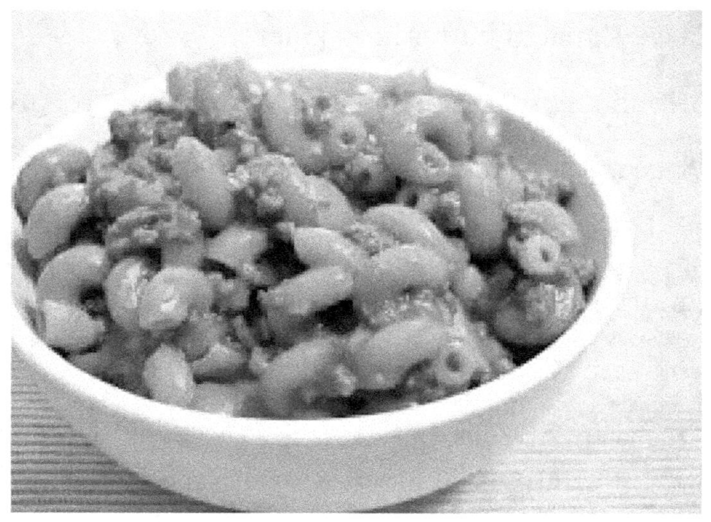

Prep time: 9 minutes

Cook time: 9 minutes

Serves: 4

Ingredients

- 1 lb ground Sirloin

- 1 chopped Onion

- 1 Chili Seasoning Mix, packet

- 1 cup tomato sauce

- 1 small can of Chunky Diced Tomatoes & Green Chilies

- 1 cup hand-shredded sharp cheddar

- 1 packet Splenda

- ½ cup Barilla Proteinplus Elbow macaroni

Directions

1. Boil Barilla Proteinplus Elbow macaroni until done, drain.

2. Brown the sirloin and onions in a large skillet.

3. Add the pasta, tomato sauce, diced tomatoes and green chilies, and chili seasoning mix.

4. Taste to see if you need to add water.

5. Serve in 4 bowls, topping each bowl with the cheddar cheese.

6. Place in four containers with lids, freeze. Microwave 2 minutes to thaw.

Nutritional Value: Calories: 480, Total Fat: 24g, Protein: 36g, Total Carbs: g, 25Dietary Fiber: 6g, Sugar: 4g, Sodium: 995mg

Seven Layer Salad

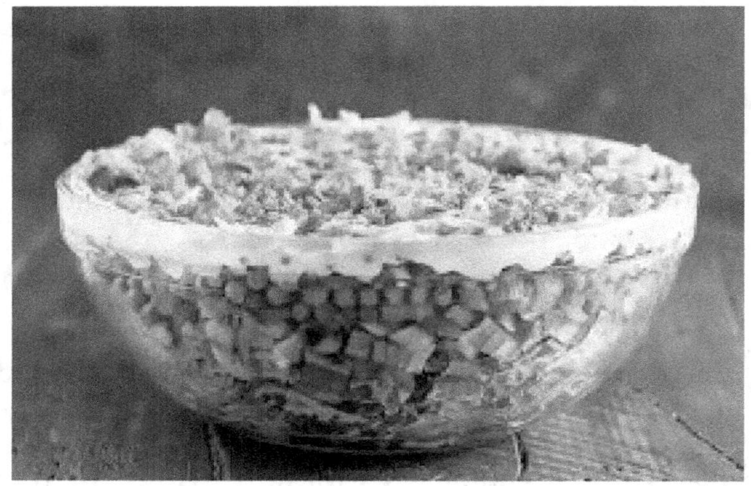

Prep time: 14 minutes

Cook time: 9 minutes

Serves: 10

Ingredients

- 4 cups shredded butter lettuce

- 4 cups shredded romaine lettuce

- 1 cup peas

- 1 cup diced bell peppers, red and yellow

- 1 cup grape tomatoes, halved

- 1 cup sliced celery

- ½ cup red onion

- ¾ cup Greek yogurt

- ¾ cup mayonnaise

- 3 hard-boiled eggs

- 2 teaspoons cider vinegar

- 1 packet Splenda

- ¼ teaspoon garlic salt

- ½ cup pepper-jack cheese, hand-shredded

- 3 strips cooked bacon, crumbled

Directions

1. Using a large glass pan, 9x13 sized, layer the two lettuces.

2. Layer the peas, then the peppers, then the tomatoes, celery and onion.

3. Place the diced eggs next.

4. Combine the dressing ingredients: yogurt, mayonnaise, vinegar, garlic salt, Splenda, and a dash of black pepper.

5. Spread the dressing over the salad.

6. Garnish with the pepper-jack cheese and bacon.

7. Place in one cup containers. Close with a lid and refrigerate.

Nutritional Value: Calories: 136, Total Fat: 7g, Protein: 2g, Total Carbs: 9g, Dietar, Fiber: 2g, Sugar: 0g, Sodium: 324mg

Chapter 11: Dinner

Healthy Kale Chicken Caesar Salad

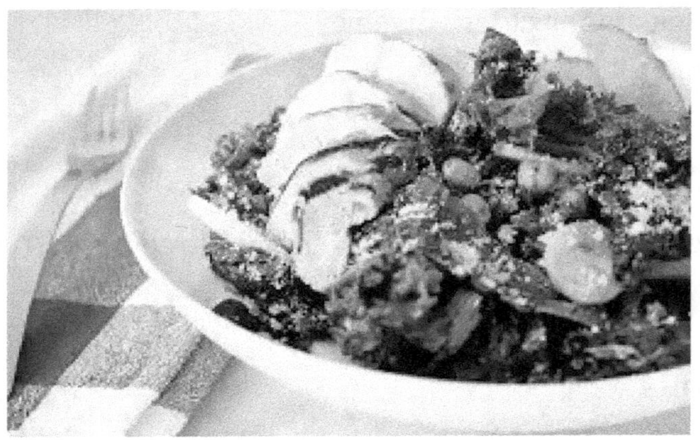

Prep Time: 35 Minutes

Serves: 8

Ingredients for the salad:

- 2 chicken breasts, boneless and skinless

- 4 tablespoon of extra virgin olive oil

- 2 tablespoon of salt

- ½ tablespoon of black pepper

- 1 tablespoon of garlic, powdered

- 1 bunch of kale, washed, chopped and with ribs removed

Ingredients for the salad dressing:

- 1 egg yolk, large

- 2 anchovies

- 1 lemon, fresh and juice only

- 1 tablespoon of apple cider

- ¼ cup of parmesan cheese, grated

- 2 tablespoon of parsley, fresh and chopped

- Dash of salt and black pepper

- ¼ cup of extra virgin olive oil

- 1 to 2 tablespoon of water

Directions:

1. First, preheat the oven to 375 degrees.

2. While the oven is heating up add the chicken breasts into a large bowl. Add in the extra virgin olive oil, dash of salt and black pepper and garlic. Toss well to mix.

3. Place the chicken breasts onto a large baking sheet. Place into the oven to bake for 30 minutes. Remove after this time and slice the chicken into thin strips.

4. Use a food processor and add in all of the ingredients for the salad dressing except for the oil. Blend on the highest setting until smooth in consistency. Then slowly pour in the oil while blending until the dressing is emulsified.

5. Place the kale in a large serving bowl. Add in the chicken and salad dressing. Toss well to mix. Serve immediately.

Nutritional Value: Calories: 208, Fat: 16 grams, Carbs: 8 grams, Protein: 8 grams

Zucchini Casserole

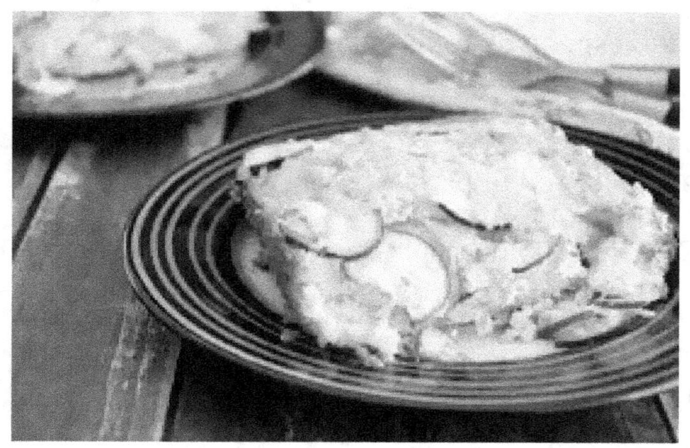

Prep Time: 1 Hour

Serves: 8

Ingredients:

- 5 pieces of bacon, chopped

- 1 onion, chopped

- 2 cloves of garlic, minced

- 2 cups of zucchini, grated

- 1 cup of Colby Jack cheese, grated

- ½ cup of almond flour

- ½ cup of vegetable oil

- ¼ cup of heavy cream

- 6 eggs, large

- Dash of salt and black pepper

Directions:

1. Place a large skillet over low to medium heat. Add in the bacon and cook for 5 minutes or until browned. Transfer the bacon to a large plate lined with paper towels to drain.

2. In the skillet with the bacon fat. Add in the onion and garlic. Stir well to mix and cook for 5 minutes or until soft. Transfer the mixture into a large bowl.

3. Add in the remaining ingredients into the bowl. Whisk well to mix and pour into a large greased baking dish.

4. Top the casserole with the shredded Colby Jack cheese.

5. Place into the oven to bake for 1 hour at 350 degrees. Make sure to turn the casserole after 30 minutes of baking.

6. Remove and allow to cool for 5 minutes before serving.

Nutritional Value: Calories: 334, Fat: 30 grams, Carbs: 6 grams, Protein: 12 grams

Oven Roasted Broccoli with Parmesan Cheese and Garlic

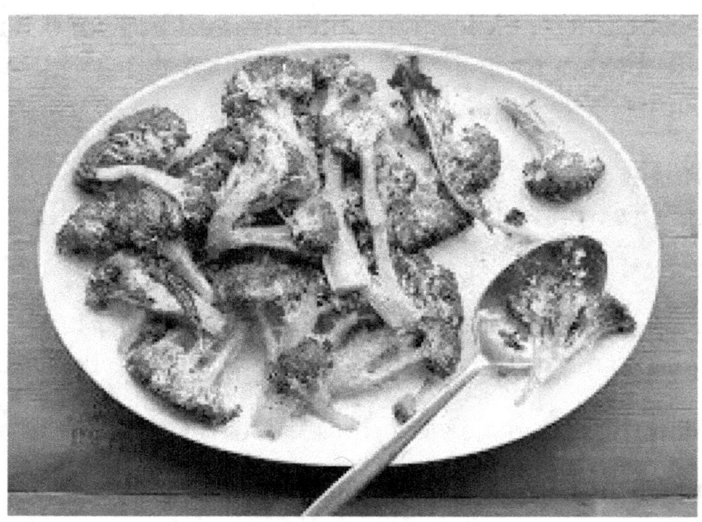

Prep Time: 20 Minutes

Serves: 4

Ingredients:

- 1 head of broccoli, fresh and cut into florets
- 2 cloves of garlic, minced
- ¼ cup of extra virgin olive oil
- Dash of salt and black pepper
- 8 tablespoon of parmesan cheese, grated and divided
- ½ of a lemon, fresh and juice only

Directions:

1. In a medium bowl add in the broccoli florets, garlic, extra virgin olive oil and dash of salt and black pepper.

2. Add in six tablespoons of the grated Parmesan cheese into the mixture and stir well to mix.

3. Add the seasoned broccoli onto a large baking sheet.

4. Place into the oven to roast at 400 degrees for 15 to 20 minutes.

5. Remove from the oven. Squeeze the fresh lemon juice over the top.

6. Sprinkle the remaining Parmesan cheese over the top and toss to coat. Serve.

Nutritional Value: Calories: 242, Fat: 18 grams, Carbs: 11 grams, Protein: 9 grams

Classic Prime Rib

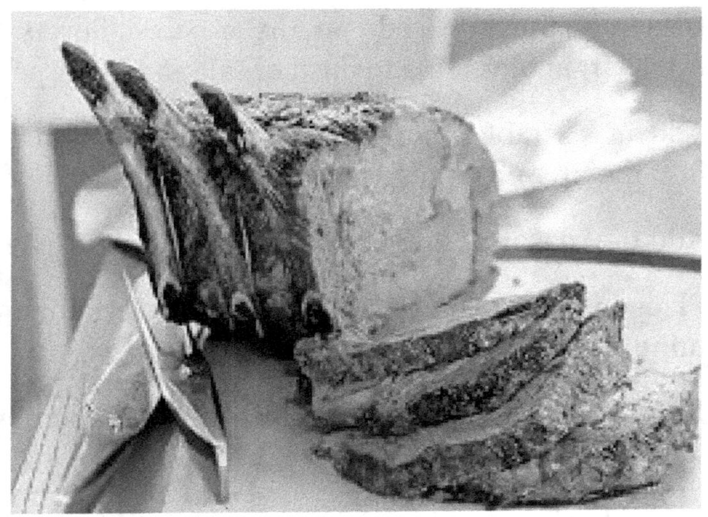

Prep Time: 3 Hours

Serves: 3

Ingredients for the prime rib:

- 1, 8 to 12 pound prime rib, boneless
- ¼ cup of extra virgin olive oil
- ½ cup of salt
- 1 tablespoon of black pepper
- 2 tablespoon of garlic, granulated
- 1 tablespoon of thyme, dried
- 1 tablespoon of rosemary, dried
- 2 tablespoon of smoked paprika

Ingredients for the horseradish cream:

- 1 cup of sour cream

- ½ cup of mayonnaise

- ¼ cup of horseradish, drained

- ½ of a lemon, juice

- Dash of Tabasco sauce

- Dash of salt and black pepper

Directions:

1. Score the skin of the prime rib with a knife.

2. Drizzle the olive oil over the prime rib. Season with: garlic, thyme, rosemary, paprika and dash of salt and black pepper.

3. Then preheat the oven to 450 to 500 degrees.

4. Place the seasoned prime rib onto a large baking sheet. Place into the oven to roast for 20 minutes. After this time increase the oven to broil and broil for another 8 minutes. Reduce the temperature of the oven to 325 degrees. Roast for 1 hour and 20 minutes.

5. Remove from the oven and set aside to rest for 30 minutes. Slice and serve.

Nutritional Value: Calories: 640, Fat: 56 grams, Carbs: 2 grams, Protein: 33 grams

Tilapia and Broccoli

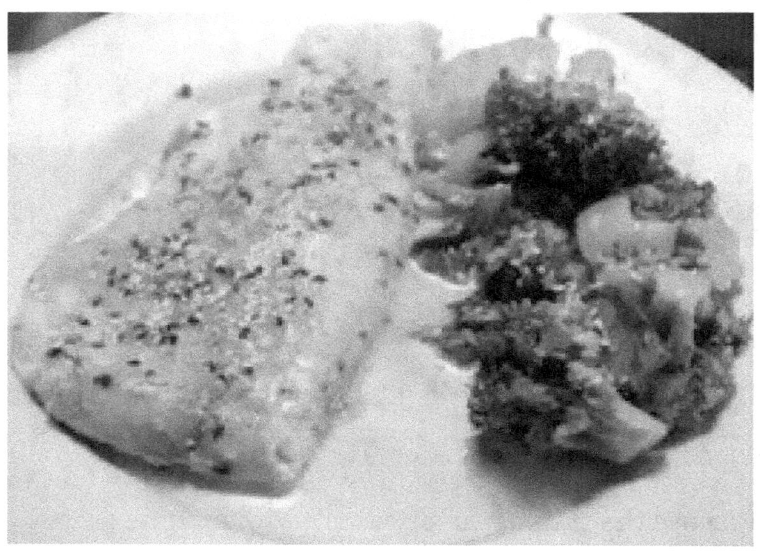

Prep time: 4 minutes

Cook time: 14 minutes

Serves: 1

Ingredients

- 6 oz. tilapia, frozen is fine

- 1 tablespoon butter

- 1 tablespoon garlic, minced or finely chopped

- 1 tablespoon of lemon pepper seasoning

- 1 cup broccoli florets, fresh or frozen, but fresh will be crisper

Directions

1. Set the pre-warmed oven for 350 degrees.

2. Place the fish in an aluminum foil packet.

3. Arrange the broccoli around the fish to make an attractive arrangement.

4. Sprinkle the lemon pepper on the fish.

5. Close the packet and seal, bake for 14 minutes.

6. Combine the garlic and butter. Set aside.

7. Remove the packet from the oven and transfer ingredients to a plate.

8. Place the butter on the fish and broccoli.

9. Place the butter and garlic into small sealed containers or zip-lock bags, Refrigerate or freeze. Cut the broccoli (if fresh) and place in zip-lock bags in the fridge. Place the lemon pepper into a small container.

Nutritional Value: Calories: 362, Total Fat: 25g, Protein: 29g, Total Carbs: 3.5g, Dietary Fiber: 3g, Sugar: 0g, Sodium: 0mg

Italian Meatballs

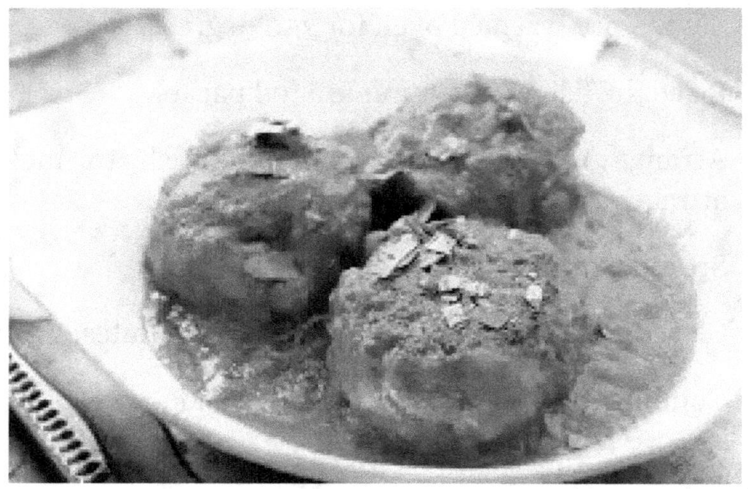

Prep Time: 40 Minutes

Serves: 4

Ingredients:

- 1 pound of beef, lean and ground

- 1 tablespoon of Italian seasoning

- 1 tablespoon of garlic, granulated

- ½ tablespoon of onion, powdered

- 2 tablespoon of salt

- ½ tablespoon of black pepper

- 1 tablespoon of Worcestershire sauce

- 2 tablespoon of tomato paste

- 1 egg, large

- 2 tablespoon of flaxseed meal

- ¼ cup of Parmesan cheese, grated

- ¼ cup of mozzarella cheese, shredded

Directions:

1. Use a large bowl and add in the ground beef, Italian seasoning, garlic, onion, a dash of salt and black pepper, Worcestershire sauce and tomato paste. Stir well to mix.

2. Add the remaining ingredients into the bowl and stir well to mix.

3. Preheat the oven to 400 degrees.

4. While the oven is heating up, form the mixture into even sized meatballs. Place the meatballs onto a lightly greased baking sheet.

5. Place into the oven to bake for 20 minutes or until cooked through.

6. Remove and serve immediately with a meal of your choice.

Nutritional Value: Calories: 451, Fat: 39 grams, Carbs: 3 grams, Protein: 22 grams

Hangar Steak

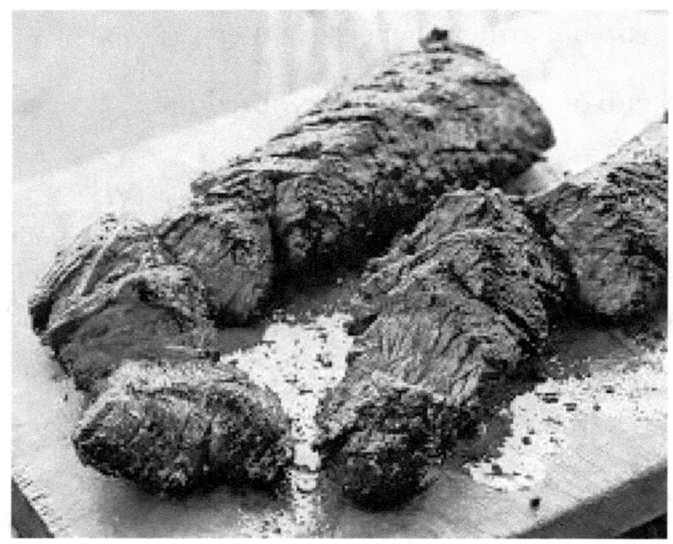

Prep Time: 4 Hours and 15 Minutes

Serves: 8

Ingredients:

- 2 pounds of hanger steak, cleaned and trimmed

- 1 tablespoon of salt

- 1 tablespoon of black pepper

- 1 tablespoon of garlic, granulated

- ½ cup of extra virgin olive

- 2 tablespoon of soy sauce

- 2 tablespoon of vinegar, red wine

- ½ cup of red wine

- 2 tablespoon of rosemary, fresh

- 1 stick of butter, melted

Directions:

1. Add all of the ingredients except for the hangar steak and melted butter into a large bowl. Stir well until evenly mixed.

2. Add in the hangar steak and toss to coat. Cover and set in the fridge to marinate for 4 hours.

3. After this time preheat an outdoor grill to medium heat.

4. Place the marinated steak onto the grill. Grill for 5 to 10 minutes on each side or until cooked to the desired doneness.

5. Remove from the grill and drizzle the melted butter over the steak. Serve.

Nutritional Value: Calories: 338, Fat: 26 grams, Carbs: 1 gram, Protein: 25 grams

Smothered Pan Seared Salmon

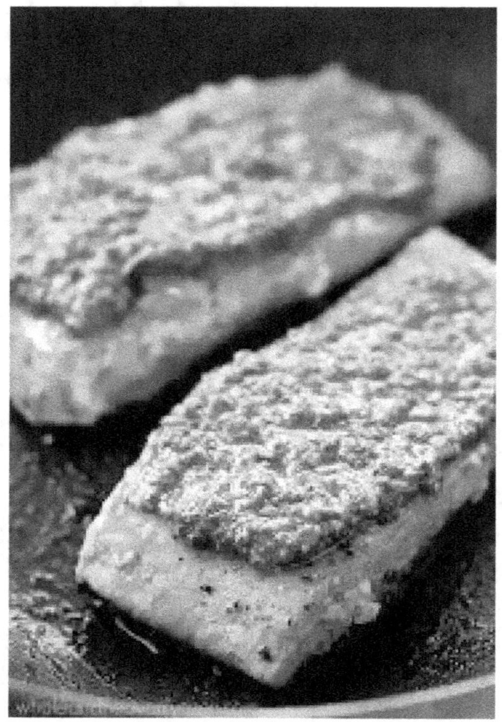

Prep Time: 20 Minutes

Serves: 4

Ingredients:

- 4, 4 ounce salmon fillets

- 2 tablespoon of coconut oil 1

- Tablespoon of salt

- ½ tablespoon of black pepper

- 1 tablespoon of garlic, powdered

- 1 tablespoon of onion, powdered

- 4 tablespoon of butter

- ½ cup of Greek yogurt, plain

- ½ cup of sour cream

- 2 tablespoon of extra virgin olive

- 1 tablespoon of dill, dried

- 1 lemon, fresh and juice only

- Dash of Tabasco sauce

Directions:

1. Use a medium bowl and add in the salt, black pepper, garlic, and onion. Stir well to mix. Sprinkle this mixture over the salmon fillets. Set the remaining seasoning aside.

2. Place a large skillet over medium to high heat. Add in the coconut oil and once the oil is hot enough add in the salmon fillets. Cook for 3 minutes on each side. Flip and continue to cook for another 3 minutes. Remove and set the salmon aside.

3. Add a tablespoon of butter over each salmon fillet.

4. Add the remaining seasoning, plain yogurt and sour cream into the skillet. Whisk until smooth in consistency. Cook for a further 2 to 3 minutes.

5. Remove from heat and pour the sauce over the top. Serve.

Nutritional Value: Calories: 558, Fat: 58 grams, Carbs: 3 grams, Protein: 24 grams

Simple Salisbury Steak

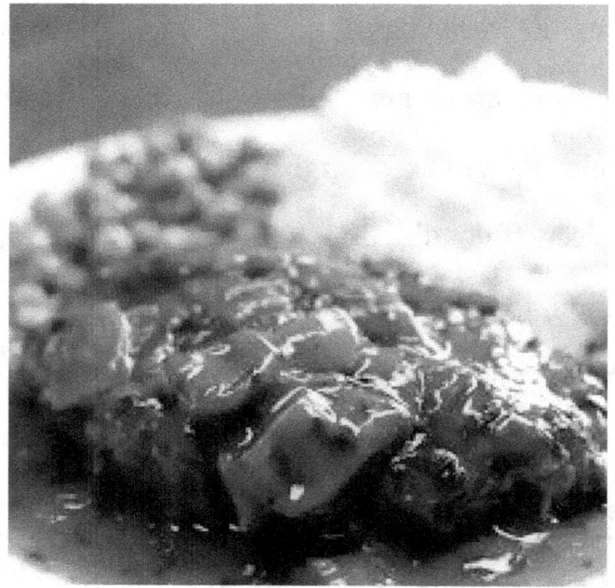

Prep Time: 20 Minutes

Serves: 8

Ingredients for the steak:

- 3 pounds of beef, lean and ground

- ½ cup of panko breadcrumbs

- 2 eggs, large

- 2 tablespoon of ketchup, low in sugar

- 4 tablespoon of mustard, dried

- 8 dashes of Worcestershire sauce

- 1 tablespoon of salt

- 1 tablespoon of black pepper

- 1 tablespoon of garlic, powdered

- 1 tablespoon of onion, powdered

- 2 tablespoon of butter

- 2 tablespoon of extra virgin olive oil

Ingredients for the gravy:

- 1 onion, sliced thinly

- 4 cups of beef broth

- 2 tablespoon of ketchup, low in sugar

- 2 tablespoon of kitchen bouquet

- 8 dashes of Worcestershire sauce

- 2 tablespoon of cornstarch

Directions:

1. Use a large bowl and add in all of the ingredients for the steak except for the butter and extra virgin olive oil. Stir well to mix and form this mixture into patties.

2. Place a large saucepan over medium heat. Add in the extra virgin olive oil and butter. As soon as the butter melts add in the beef patties. Cook for 8 minutes on each side or until cooked through.

3. Remove the cooked patties from the skillet and transfer to a large plate.

4. Add the sliced onions into the skillet. Cook for 5 to 10 minutes or until soft.

5. Then add in the beef broth, low sugar ketchup, kitchen bouquet and Worcestershire sauce. Whisk until smooth in consistency.

6. Add in the cornstarch and whisk to mix. Continue to cook for an additional 2 minutes or until thick in consistency.

7. Add the cooked patties into the gravy and toss to mix.

8. Remove from heat and serve.

Nutritional Value: Calories: 519, Fat: 59 grams, Carbs: 18 grams, Protein: 29 grams

Chapter 12: Desserts and Appetizers

Chocolate Truffles

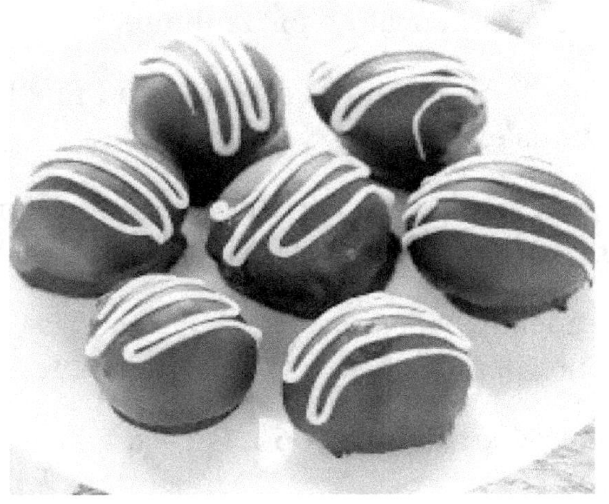

Preparation time: 10 minutes

Cooking time: 6 minutes

Servings: 22

Ingredients:

- 1 cup sugar-free chocolate chips

- 2 tablespoons butter

- ⅔ cup heavy cream

- 2 teaspoons brandy

- 2 tablespoons swerve

- ¼ teaspoon vanilla extract

- Cocoa powder

Directions:

1. Put the heavy cream in a heatproof bowl, add the swerve, butter, and chocolate chips, stir, introduce in a microwave, and heat up for 1 minute.

2. Set aside for 5 minutes, stir well, and mix with brandy, and vanilla extract.

3. Stir again and set aside in the refrigerator for a couple of hours.

4. Use a melon baller to shape the truffles, roll them in cocoa powder, and serve.

Nutritional Value: Calories - 60, Fat - 5, Fiber - 4, Carbs - 6, Protein - 1

Doughnuts

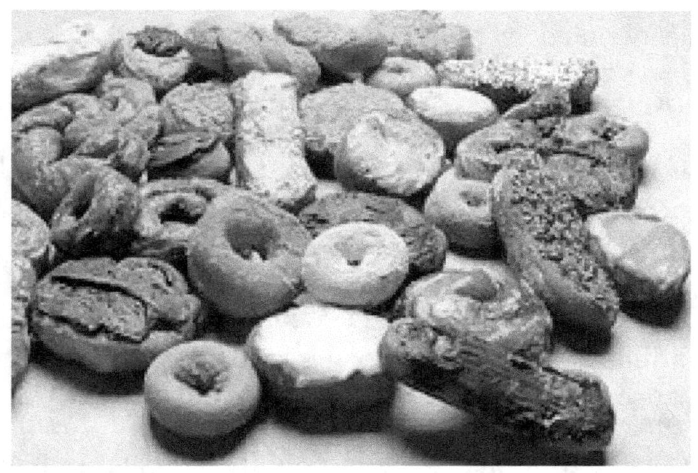

Preparation time: 10 minutes

Cooking time: 15 minutes

Servings: 24

Ingredients:

- ¼ cup erythritol

- ¼ cup flaxseed meal

- ¾ cup almond flour

- 1 teaspoon baking powder

- 1 teaspoon vanilla extract

- 2 eggs

- 3 tablespoons coconut oil

- ¼ cup coconut milk

- 20 drops red food coloring

- A pinch of salt

- 1 tablespoon cocoa powder

Directions:

1. In a bowl, mix the flaxseed meal with almond flour, cocoa powder, baking powder, erythritol, and salt, and stir.

2. In another bowl, mix the coconut oil with coconut milk, vanilla extract, food coloring, and eggs, and stir.

3. Combine the 2 mixtures, stir using a hand mixer, transfer to a bag, make a hole in the bag, and shape 12 doughnuts on a baking sheet.

4. Place in an oven at 350°F, and bake for 15 minutes. Arrange them on a platter and serve.

Nutritional Value: Calories - 60, Fat - 4, Fiber - 0, Carbs - 1, Protein - 2

Chocolate Bombs

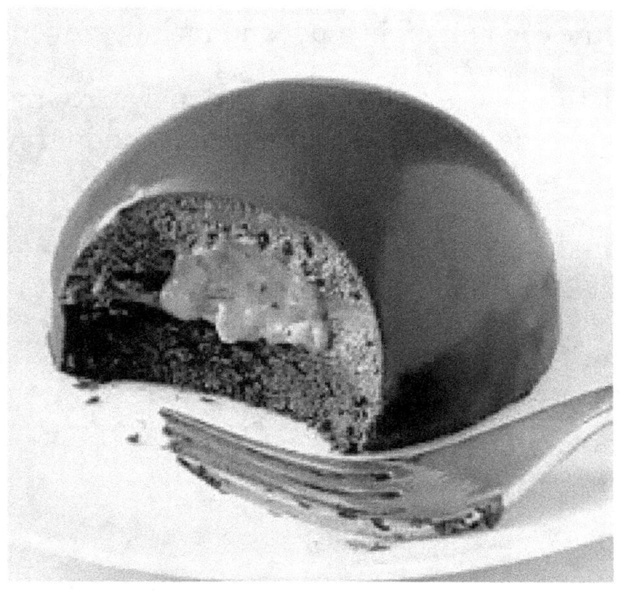

Preparation time: 10 minutes

Cooking time: 10 minutes

Servings: 12

Ingredients:

- 10 tablespoons coconut oil

- 3 tablespoons macadamia nuts, chopped

- 2 packets stevia

- 5 tablespoons unsweetened coconut powder

- A pinch of salt

Directions:

1. Put the coconut oil in a pot and melt over medium heat.

2. Add the stevia, salt, and cocoa powder, stir well, and take off the heat. Spoon this into a candy tray and keep in the refrigerator for a couple of hours.

3. Sprinkle the macadamia nuts on top, and keep in the refrigerator until ready to serve.

Nutritional Value: Calories - 50, Fat - 1, Fiber - 0, Carbs - 1, Protein - 2

Kale Crackers

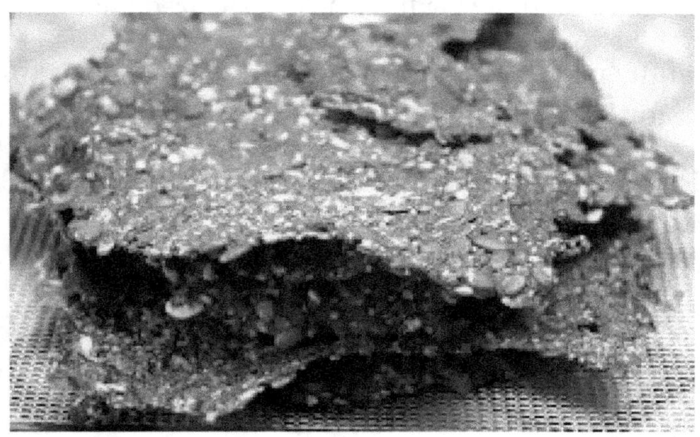

Ingredients

- 3 tablespoons Filtered Water

- ½ cup Fresh Kale, trimmed and chopped

- ½ cup, plus 2 tablespoons, Whole Wheat Flour

- ½ teaspoon Dried Rosemary, crushed

- Pinch of Himalayan Pink Salt

- Pinch of Red Pepper Flakes, crushed

- 2 tablespoons Almond Butter

Directions

1.   Preheat the oven to 400 degrees F and line a large baking sheet with parchment paper.

2.   In a blender, add the water and kale and pulse until smooth. In a bowl, mix the flour, rosemary, salt and red pepper flakes. Add the butter and mix until the mixture becomes crumbly. Stir in the kale mixture and mix until dough forms.

Roll the dough into a thin layer on a floured smooth surface. Cut the rolled dough according to your desired shape.

3. Carefully place the crackers onto the prepared baking sheet and bake for 8 to 10 minutes.

Nutritional Value: Calories: 338, Fat: 26 grams, Carbs: 1 gram, Protein: 25 grams

Conclusion

The first stage of the diet, called induction or stimulating, is necessary for the conversion of human metabolism to ketosis (Ketosis). With ketosis, the body produces ketones from fat cells to produce energy in the tricarboxylic acid cycle, the Krebs cycle. That is, the Atkins diet is ketogenic. Such diets can improve the regulation of insulin in the blood, which is especially important for type 2 diabetes mellitus because people on a ketogenic diet at little carbohydrates, a significant amount of glucose is not formed in the blood for the release of insulin. Since there is no glucose-insulin reaction, changes in metabolic processes occur in the body, leading to the use of accumulated fat cells for energy.

The blood glucose level decreases to values less than 3.58 mmol/l (a pathological condition called hypoglycemia), in which the body produces growth hormone, adrenaline and hyperglycemic pancreatic hormone (glucagon) to maintain metabolism. In adipose tissue cell growth hormones and adrenaline activate the mechanisms of cleavage of triacylglycerol into fatty acids. These fatty acids enter the muscle tissue and liver, where they are oxidized and form acetyl-CoA, which directly enters the Krebs cycle.

The excess of acetyl-CoA in the liver is converted to ketones (ketone bodies), which are secreted by the liver and subsequently converted again in the muscles and brain back to acetyl-CoA to enter the Krebs cycle. Glucagon is produced only at low blood glucose levels and initiates the liver breakdown of glycogen into glucose. If a person's carbohydrate intake remains low, glycogen levels in the liver, it begins to break down fats into free fatty acids and ketone bodies, a process called ketosis. Accordingly, the Atkins diet is a type of ketogenic diet.

Reference

https://www.atkins.com/

https://www.atkins.com/

https://www.healthline.com/nutrition/atkins-diet-101